NURSING CARE OF THE
HEMIPLEGIC STROKE PATIENT

NURSING CARE OF THE HEMIPLEGIC STROKE PATIENT

Freda Myco BA, SRN, BTA cert, RNT
Lecturer in Nursing Studies
New University of Ulster

Harper & Row, Publishers
London

Cambridge		San Francisco
Hagerstown		Mexico City
Philadelphia		Sao Paulo
New York		Sydney

First published 1983

Harper & Row Ltd
28 Tavistock Street
London WC2E 7PN

British Library Cataloguing in Publication Data

Myco, Freda
    Nursing care of the hemiplegic stroke patient.
    1. Hemiplegics—Nursing
    I. Title
    610.73'8   RC406.H45

    ISBN 0-06-318248-3

Typeset by Gedset, Cheltenham.
Printed by Butler and Tanner, Frome, Somerset.

To 'Ollie'
for his advice and support

CONTENTS

PREFACE

Sheer facts are not knowledge. It is the pattern of successful organization of facts that is central to knowledge. The acquisition of knowledge in an organized way is essential for the nurse who seeks to make her* observations adequate for the assessment of the dependency-needs level of a stroke patient. Such an assessment enables the nurse to determine the patient's problems, establish priorities, and develop a plan of care in coordination with other team members.

It is not the aim of this book to present an extensive reiteration of the wide array of knowledge concerning singular aspects of stroke which are well described by other authors. Such information sources are indicated by reference and bibliography. Rather it attempts to concentrate on that material which can be considered as being fundamental to the nurse's role in stroke patient care in both hospital and community. The nurse caring for the stroke patient needs to acquire a greater depth of knowledge as a platform for developing philosophy and skill. The nurse should:

1 Increase her level of knowledge of anatomy, physiology and pathology of the main systems concerned, namely the nervous, musculo-skeletal and urinary systems.
2 Know some basic facts about kinesiology, the science of movement.

---

*For purposes of simplification, the nurse is given the female gender and the patient the male gender throughout the book.

3 Develop understanding of the psychological problems of long-term disability so as to be able to support the patient at each appropriate stage.

4 Have a working knowledge of the reasons for faecal and urinary incontinence, and the ways by which a patient can be helped to regain control.

5 Understand why stroke patients can have difficulty explaining their needs and understanding others, so as to be able to establish some method of communication.

6 Know what services are available for the patient and his family in their community, including spiritual support.

7 Understand, and build into the care process, ways by which the patient may adjust to the socio-economic effects of his environment and circumstances.

The author assumes the reader has a basic understanding of the structure and function of the health and personal social services, the elements of the nursing process, the anatomy and physiology of the systems concerned, as well as the theories of accepted psycho-social norms.

The text of the book is divided into three unequal sections. An introduction deals with the basic epidemiology, aetiology and clinical manifestations of stroke. The second section describes the care of the patient in the early stages of post-stroke recovery. The final and largest section discusses the long-term rehabilitative care required by stroke patients, and these chapters are organized within the framework of principles of nursing care postulated by Henderson (1967).

Much of the disability suffered by stroke victims can be obviated by the early application of rehabilitative care. Thereby the nurse caring for these patients can receive a great deal of satisfaction from knowing that by careful planning with the patient, his family and other health personnel, she is capable of preventing physical deterioration as well as loss of dignity and the misery often suffered by these patients. The author hopes this book might help to bring about such satisfaction.

Reference

Henderson, V (1967) Basic Principles of Nursing Care, ICN

INTRODUCTION

'Stroke victims cry softly in their need. Often nurses do not hear them above the din of seemingly more demanding and exciting things that must be done' (McNeil 1975). The compendium of miseries that a person who has had a stroke may have to endure has been aptly summed up as, 'being treated like an idiot, to be ignored or to be shouted at; the frustration of having things done for him which were well within his own capacity; even worse, the failure to foresee and do things he could not possibly do for himself; and being kept in bed when he longed to be up . . .' (Adams 1972).

The first consistent contact that a stroke patient makes with the health services after his catastrophe is with the nurse. What she does, how she approaches the patient, her attitude and her insights may be directly responsible for the type of recovery the patient is to enjoy (Wepman 1951). While medical and paramedical services may be available and may play an important role in therapeusis, the patient spends most of his time directly with the nurse. Consequently, the largest share of the care burden lies, and will continue to lie, with her. In stroke the indications for medical or surgical intervention remain few (Whisnant 1977). In addition, attempts to improve the prognosis of stroke by providing intensive care facilities have proved unsuccessful (Kennedy et al. 1970). Following a report by the Royal College of Physicians in 1974, a few specialized rehabilitation units were set up in large city areas (Working group on strokes 1974). However, access to such centres is normally by referral which necessarily involves selection, usually based on the stroke victim's initial prognosis (Isaacs 1977).

Therefore, for the majority of stroke victims it will remain the responsibility of the nurse to set the tone of the recovery process, whether in hospital or in the home. Competent nursing of these patients makes it mandatory that the nurse be carefully informed regarding the cause of the stroke and the possible complications that may develop; factors which must be considered in the planning of patient care (Schultz 1968). Lack of such information can lead to overprotectiveness by the nurse so that months, sometimes years after his initial admission the patient is still languishing in an early stage of recovery.

Authors differ in their claims regarding the anticipated period of optimum recovery from stroke. According to Tool and Patel (1974), the neurologic deficit from infarction reaches its peak within the first 72 hours. Some improvement may be apparent after the first 2 weeks, with maximum recovery in most cases by 22 weeks. No further recovery, they claim, should be expected after 6-9 months. While some authors support 6 months as the point of maximum recovery (e.g. diBenedetto 1974), others put it closer to 3 months, (e.g. Kurasick and Sutton 1969). However, Adams (1974) claims that recovery often takes 2 years.

The size of the problem

The populations of industrialized societies are growing older. In Britain 16% of the population is over 65 years of age, and this percentage is likely to increase to nearly 20% by the end of the century (McGilloway 1979). As the majority of stroke victims are 65 years or over, stroke is a major burden on the community (WHO 1971). In one study the median age of 383 cases of stroke was 73 years (Gibson 1974), but the minimum range is steadily falling and more victims can be found in the 50 year old group, and occasionally even younger. Stroke has now become the third most frequent cause of death in most developed countries, being exceeded only by heart disease and cancer.

The annual incidence rate in Britain, and the USA, is said to be just under 2/1000 of the population (Brewis et al. 1966, Hurwitz and Adams 1972, Matsumoto et al. 1973, Isaacs 1977 and Marshall 1979). Some earlier studies of localized populations in these countries placed the annual frequency rate closer to 3% of the population (Kannelin 1966, Larrson 1967). However, the exact incidence cannot be pinpointed because no truly representative statistics are kept. The incidence of stroke appears to rise sharply in relation to increasing age, and sex. Studies in Sweden, Denmark and the USA claim that up to 40 years of age the morbidity risk of stroke in the population is only 0.1%, but that this doubles over each consecutive 5 year period until, by 90 years, it reaches 45% (Marquardsen 1969, Whisnant et al. 1971 and Eisenberg et al. 1964). As females tend to live longer than males in most Western societies, the ratio of strokes between males and females over 65 years rests in the favour of females.

International studies appear to agree that about 50% of stroke victims die in the first 2-3 weeks following their catastrophe; usually in the first few days (Marquardsen 1969, Geltner 1972 and Wu Ying Kai 1979). However, there are some international differences in incidence and mortality rates. For example, in China and Japan stroke incidence and mortality rates tend to be higher than in Europe and North America (Takahashi et al. 1961, Kannelin 1966). As well as demographic factors, various conditions are claimed as increasing the risk of stroke. Hypertension and diabetes mellitus head most lists (WHO 1971, Acheson and Hutchinson 1971). Yet despite such widespread awareness that hypertension is a major cause of stroke, the World Health Organization claims that control of this condition is, in general, far from satisfactory in most countries.

In terms of actual numbers of stroke victims surviving in Britain, a survey for the Office of Populations, Censuses and Surveys estimated there were 130 000 persons with this form of handicap living in private households, in 1971. In 93 000 of these cases, the disability was severe or very serious (Harris et al. 1971). In the USA, the disability level has been put at 2 million people (Policoff 1970). Extrapolation from these figures to a population of 250 000 (the basis for a district general hospital in Britain) would suggest an incidence of 500 stroke victims each year, of which 250 will need a lot of help and about 150 of these will be added each year to the accumulating number needing continued care (Hurwitz and Adams 1972).

Such statistics are likely to continue to increase for the foreseeable future as the population becomes more elderly, while stroke prevention techniques are still in their infancy (Joint Committee for Stroke Facilities 1972).

What is stroke?

The World Health Organization states, 'a stroke is characterised by a focal neurological deficit due to a local disturbance in the blood supply to the brain: its onset is usually abrupt but may extend over a few hours or longer' (WHO 1971).

The causes of stroke are many (Table 1). Whatever the cause, however, it is important to remember that the nervous system has a limited pathological and functional response to disease and catastrophe. An isolated lesion in either

Table 1 The causes of stroke

Arteriosclerosis (atheroma)

Embolism

Congenital abnormalities of blood vessels, e.g. malformation or aneurysm

Tumour, e.g. benign or malignant, primary or secondary

Trauma

Infection of the blood vessels:
  (a) primary, e.g. arteritis
  (b) secondary, e.g. meningitis, encephalitis

Systemic disease, e.g. hypertension, syphilis, eclampsia, leukaemia and a variety of infectious diseases

---

hemisphere of the brain will give rise to a hemiparesis (weakness), or hemiplegia (paralysis), on the opposite side of the body. If the lesion becomes settled and chronic the same rehabilitative principles and techniques are used irrespective of aetiology.

The three most frequent causes of hemiplegic stroke are thrombosis, haemorrhage and embolism. Kurtze (1969) reviewed over four hundred original papers on cerebrovascular epidemiology up to 1967. He estimated the causes of death from stroke in 18 countries, including Britain, after allowing for the variation in ways of classifying data, as being:

Cause	Percentage of deaths
Cerebral thrombosis	62
Cerebral haemorrhage	16
Subarachnoid haemorrhage	12
Embolism and other causes	10

Other authors claim that intravascular thrombosis, caused by the accumulation of fatty deposits in the lumen of blood vessels leading to total occlusion, is even more common, accounting for 80% of strokes (Millikan 1964, Kurasik and Sutton 1969).

There would appear to be two distinct groups of patients who present with strokes — those whose life is punctuated by recurring attacks leading to an early death, and those who have fewer attacks and survive many years (Marshall and Shaw 1959). The difference may be attributable to the presence, or otherwise, of hypertension (Acheson and Hutchinson 1971).

All strokes do not develop at the same rate; some develop over several minutes or hours, others have a very abrupt onset without any immediate or premonitory symptoms (Marshall 1976). Some strokes occur while the patient is asleep. This might be caused by alterations in intravascular pressure brought about by positional change. Some strokes of rapid onset have an equally rapid recovery. For example, transient ischaemic attacks (TIAs) can come on abruptly, but persist for only minutes or hours, before clearing completely. A TIA is generally defined as an attack which clears up within 24 hours. They are usually associated with disease of the walls of the carotid arteries. A 'stroke-in-evolution' is one which develops slowly, taking at least 6 hours to reach its peak, while a 'completed stroke' comes on acutely, in less than 6 hours, and thereafter persists.

Following a stroke, life expectancy is affected by the age of the person, the severity of any preceding hypertension, or any accompanying cardiac dysfunction, and the duration and depth of initial unconsciousness. Probably few of the patients whose cerebral haemorrhage is attributable to hypertension survive to make good recoveries. About one in three stroke patients with cerebral haemorrhage die within 3 months, and a further third within 3 years (Nichols 1976). Given that the prognosis of the outcome of stroke rests on the interplay of factors individual to one patient, a study of the resultant prognosis of 710 hospital patients, who survived the initial shock of stroke, showed the following results. 19% died within 2 months of onset, 39% were confined to bed, confused and incontinent, and 42% recovered overall. Those who recovered were divided into two categories of approximately half each. The first of these categories (about 20% of the overall number) were fully independent, had some use of their hand, walked confidently and had a clear intellect. The second category of recovery contained those who needed help with walking, had some overall handicap, and some mental clouding. They represented 20% of the overall number (Adams and Merrett 1961). Remember these numbers do not include those who died at the onset of the stroke. The survivors for the most part are those whose strokes are caused by occlusion due to atheroma, i.e. cerebral thrombosis (Adams 1974). In cases of occlusion, the blood supply carrying oxygen, glucose and other nutrients to the brain cells is cut off from the part of the brain served by the affected artery (Figure 0.1). An infarction is said to have occurred. Without oxygen the brain tissue dies, and the bodily function controlled by that area of the brain is diminished or permanently lost, depending on the amount of brain tissue involved.

Diagram to show cerebral circulation

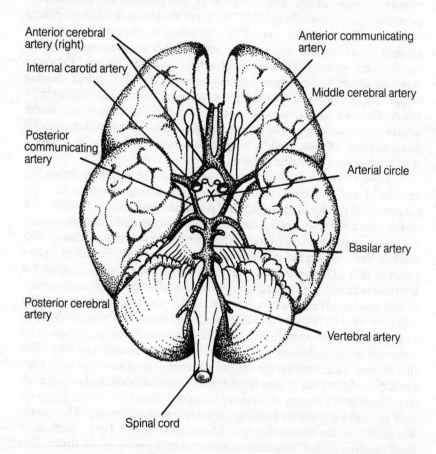

Anterior cerebral artery (right)

Internal carotid artery

Posterior communicating artery

Posterior cerebral artery

Spinal cord

Anterior communicating artery

Middle cerebral artery

Arterial circle

Basilar artery

Vertebral artery

Clinical manifestations

The signs and symptoms, or clinical manifestations, of stroke are infinitely variable, depending on which artery, large or small, and consequently which area of the brain is affected. Subsequent recovery of function depends on whether or not a collateral circulation can be rapidly established, and what amount of dysfunction in the initial stage might be caused by cerebral oedema.

Within the limitations of diagnosis, the symptoms attributable to occlusion of the major arteries supplying the brain have been described as follows (Bannister 1973, Adams 1974 and Levenson 1978).

Internal carotid artery

The patient often complains of having warning attacks of blindness in one eye, and motor and sensory impairment on one side of his body. Such transient attacks increase until a more serious attack, accompanied by confusion or unconsciousness, occurs, leaving the patient with loss of function (hemiplegia), loss of feeling or sensory ability (hemianaesthesia), and loss of vision (hemianopia), on the affected side. While most functional and sensory centres are duplicated, i.e. one centre in each hemisphere of the brain, there is only one main centre for speech or language. This is usually located in the opposite hemisphere to the patient's dominant side. For example, a right-handed person is said to be right-side dominant, and his language centre will be located on the left side of his brain. If this side is seriously affected the patient will exhibit both expressive and receptive aphasia, i.e. he will not be able to understand what is being said to him or make himself understood verbally.

Because there is a good chance that a collateral or by-pass circulation can be established, recovery is possible and residual dysfunction is unpredictable. The nurse can expect a varied range of signs and symptoms from patients with carotid involvement (Groch, Hurwitz and McDowell 1960). Frequent and detailed assessments should be made on these patients as their health status can fluctuate rapidly. The nurse-in-charge might find it useful to encourage all staff to make a brief note on their transactions with this patient, thereby increasing the accuracy of the daily summary of his needs. Small, yet important, changes or warnings might be noted which would otherwise go unrecorded and unheeded in the hustle and bustle of the day.

Middle cerebral artery

This artery is a branch of the internal carotid. Disruption of blood flow results in hemiplegia on the opposite side, especially affecting the face, tongue and arm. Consequently, the patient's ability to swallow and to conduct activities such as dressing will be hampered. Because the leg is usually less involved the outlook for regaining mobility is good.

The nearer the occlusion is to the artery's origin at the internal carotid, the less opportunity there is for a collateral circulation to be developed, and the more intense will be the clinical picture of hemiplegia, sensory loss and one-sided visual disturbance. The more distal the occlusion, i.e. further away from the source of the artery, the more likely it will be that the language centre will escape impairment, if it is in the damaged side of the brain.

Anterior cerebral artery

Following occlusion of this artery, the lower extremity tends to be affected more than the arm. Sensory and functional loss in the leg are both apparent. The arm may exhibit spastic, involuntary or reflex movements. Aphasia (language impairment), and apraxia (forgetting simple, learned activities) may occur. Incontinence of urine is sometimes persistent in these patients despite recovery in other respects, and this is often accompanied by a strange lack of concern about the social consequences (Adams 1974).

Basilar artery

The basilar artery, which is formed from the two vertebral arteries, nourishes ten of the twelve cranial nerves and several vital centres, including the brain stem. It also nourishes all the ascending and descending tracts, and the organs of balance and hearing. The symptoms, many and varied, are usually cata-strophic, and the outcome is usually rapidly fatal if the main branch is occluded, i.e. before the artery divides. There is usually a rapid loss of con-sciousness, Cheyne-Stokes respiration, small fixed pupils, severe impairment of the swallowing reflex, difficulty in moving limbs, and tremors or palsy-like movements.

Posterior cerebral arteries

These two arteries arise from the bifurcation of the basilar artery. They supply various parts of the middle and rear portions of the brain, including the thala-mus, internal capsule, and the cortex of the temporal and occipital lobes. As these parts of the brain have various specific functions the symptoms will depend on which part is affected by the infarction. There is sometimes visual disturbance on the opposite side accompanied by a lack of awareness that the visual field has been obliterated. This is called visual agnosia (what is on the affected side is not seen and therefore does not exist). Contralateral hemi-plegia, spontaneous pain and palsied movements sometimes occur.

    Occipital lobe involvement with progressive atheroma can lead to gradual or sudden blindness. Confusion is common when the posterior cerebral arteries are involved, and the mortality rate is high.

Hemisphere-related manifestations

Patients with infarction of the non-dominant hemisphere leading to severe residual hemiplegia and hemianopia often fail to admit that they have anything wrong with the affected side (anosognosia). This is particularly so in the early weeks following their catastrophe. They may offer a bizarre reason for the paralysis or even disown the paralyzed side altogether. This has implications for the nursing care plan. A voice from the patient's blind side will have no obvious source and might therefore be ignored by the patient. It is sometimes difficult for junior nurses to appreciate that when approaching these patients on the wrong side they might get no response, they do not 'exist' for the patient and nothing is happening in the patient's awareness even though the nurse might be touching him on the affected arm.

The patient with right-hemisphere damage, especially of the parietal lobe, might exhibit perceptual deficits. In most people this hemisphere appears to be responsible for perception, i.e. how we see our personal world, an ability acquired in the first 10 years of life (Penfield 1966). The patient will be disorientated, and unable to manipulate the components of his environment so as to get about in his normal way, even when in familiar surroundings. These patients tend to lose their sense of position in space and their knowledge of the geographical layout of their world, for example which is their bed or where the toilet is located despite having been there many times, or they might fail to recognize the street or even the house where they have lived all their lives. They forget how to dress, trying to put a coat on backwards or pull trousers over their heads. They fail to recognize familiar faces. Their activities are carried out too quickly to be efficient. If the patient is elderly, such disturbances can easily be mistaken for dementia. The nurse should ask relatives and friends about how the patient could cope with everyday activities before the stroke to avoid such a mistake occurring.

These patients can usually understand oral or written instructions but demonstrations confuse them. When asked to draw or copy a common object, or a scene of activity, the drawing will tend to be rigid and full of omissions not usually expected from adults.

Because the left hemisphere appears to involve the conceptual area of logic, analysis and ideas, infarction here may lead to a very slow task performance by the patient when asked to do something by the nurse or occupational therapist. This patient may have difficulty with oral or written instructions, but understand demonstrations quite well.

The nurse who is aware of the location of the patient's infarction or haemorrhage will be able to observe the patient more accurately for the range of anticipated disabilities and perceptual disturbances. Without such observations any assessment and, therefore, care plan will be incomplete. Perhaps the most unfortunate thing that can happen when a nurse has limited knowledge about what a stroke is, is that it can arouse an attitude of hopelessness stemming from ignorance rather than knowledge, unknowingly depriving the patient of proper assistance (Stryker 1972).

References

Acheson, J and Hutchinson, E C (1971) The natural history of focal cerebral vascular disease, Quarterly Journal of Medicine, 40: 15-23

Adams, G F (1972) Principles of the treatment of stroke, Nursing Mirror, 141 (35): 12

Adams, G F (1974) Cerebral Vascular Disability and the Ageing Brain, Churchill Livingstone

Adams, G F and Merrett, J D (1961) Prognosis and survival after strokes, British Medical Journal, 1: 309-314

Bannister, R (1973) Brain's Clinical Neurology, 4th edition, Oxford University Press, pp 218-31

Brewis, M, Poskanzer, D C, Rolland, C and Miller, H (1966) Neurological disease in an English city, Acta Neurologica Scandinavica, 42: 10-89

diBenedetto, M (1974) Optimal care for the severely impaired stroke patient, Rehabilitation (London), 91, Oct-Dec: 27-35

Eisenberg, H, Morrison, J T, Sullivan, P and Foote, F M (1964) Cerebral vascular accidents, Journal of the American Medical Association, 189:883-888

Geltner, K (1972) Comprehensive care of cerebral vascular accidents, Gerontologica Clinica, 14: 346-353

Gibson, C D (1974) Epidemiology and patterns of care of stroke patients, Archives of Physical Medical Rehabilitation, 55, Sept: 398-403

Groch, S N, Hurwitz, L and McDowell, F (1960) Bilateral carotid artery occlusive disease, Archives of Neurology, 12: 130-133

Harris, A I, Cox, E and Smith, C R W (1971) Handicapped and Impaired in Great Britain, Office of Populations, Censuses and Surveys, HMSO

Hurwitz, L J and Adams, G F (1972) Rehabilitation of hemiplegia — indices of assessment and prognosis, British Medical Journal, 1: 94-98

Isaacs, B (1977) Five years experience of a stroke unit, Health Bulletin (Edinburgh), 35: 94-98

Joint Committee for Stroke Facilities (1972) Report Number 5 — Clinical prevention of stroke, Stroke 3: 804-825

Kannelin, B (1966) Report of the 5th conference of cerebral vascular disease, volume 53

Kennedy, F B, Pozen, T J and Bagelman, E H (1970) Stroke intensive care — an appraisal, American Heart Journal, 180: 188-196

Kurasik, S and Sutton, B B (1969) Management of the hemiplegic stroke patient, Journal of the American Geriatrics Society, 17, July: 701-709

Kurtze, J F (1969) Epidemiology of Cerebrovascular Disease, Springer-Verlag

Larrson, T (1967) Thule International Symposia, volume 15

Levenson, C (1978) Rehabilitation of the stroke hemiplegic patient, in Krusen, Kottke and Ellwood (eds), Handbook of Rehabilitation Medicine, 2nd edition, W B Saunders

McGilloway, F A (1979) Care of the elderly — a national and international issue, Journal of Advanced Nursing, 4 (5): 545-555

McNeil, F (1975) Stroke — nursing insights from a stroke-nurse victim, Registered Nurse, 38, Sept: 75-81

Marquardsen, J (1969) The natural history of acute cerebrovascular accident — a retrospective study of 769 patients (1940-1952), Acta Neurologica Scandinavica, 45, Supplement: 38

Marshall, D (1979) MRC annual report 1978-9 — a brief guide to the report, Health Trends, 11 (4): 81

Marshall, J (1976) The Management of Cerebrovascular Accident, 3rd edition, Blackwell Scientific Publications

Marshall, J and Shaw, D A (1959) The natural history of cerebral vascular disease, British Medical Journal, 1: 1614-1617

Matsumoto, N, Whisnant, J P, Kurland, L T and Okazaki, H (1973) Natural history of stroke in Rochester, Minnesota — 1959-1969; an extension of a previous study, 1945-1954, Stroke, 4: 20-29

Millikan, C H (1964) Diagnosis of the stroke-prone patient, in R E DeForest (Editor) Proceedings of the National Stroke Congress, Charles C Thomas

Nichols, P J R (1976) Rehabilitation Medicine — the Management of Physical Disabilities, Butterworths

Penfield, W (1966) Speech, perception and the uncommitted cortex, in J C Eccles, (Editor) Brain and Conscious Experience, Springer-Verlag

Policoff, L D (1970) The philosophy of stroke rehabilitation, Geriatrics, 25 March: 99-107

Schultz, L C M (1968) The nursing care of a patient with stroke, Alabama Journal of Medical Science, 5, Jan: 27-33

Stryker, R P (1972) Rehabilitative Aspects of Acute and Chronic Nursing Care, W B Saunders

Takahashi, E, Kato, K, Kawakama, Y, Ishiguro, K, Kaneta, S, Kobayashi, S, Ohba, E, Yano, S, Ito, Y, Shiraishi, M, Murakami, N, Sugawara, T, Megure, Y and Suzuki, Y (1961) Epidemiological studies on hypertension and cerebral haemorrhage in north-east Japan, Tohoku Journal of Experimental Medicine, 74 (2): 188-210

Tool, J F and Patel, A N (1974) Cerebral Vascular Disorders, McGraw-Hill

Wepman, J M (1951) Recovery from Aphasia, Ronald Press

Whishnant, J P (1977) Indications for medical and surgical therapy for ischaemic stroke, in R A Thompson and J R Green (Editors) Advances in Neurology, Raven Press, 16: 133-144

Whishnant, J P, Fitzgibbons, J P, Kurland, L T and Sayre, G P (1971) Natural history of stroke in Rochester, Minnesota 1945-1954, Stroke 2: 11-22

World Health Organization (1971a) Cerebrovascular diseases — prevention, treatment and rehabilitation, Technical report service no 469, WHO

World Health Organization (1971b) Stroke — treatment, rehabilitation and prevention, WHO Chronicle, 25, Oct: 466-469

Working group on strokes (1974) Report of the Geriatric Committee of the Royal College of Physicians

Wu Ying Kai (1979) Epidemiology and community control of hypertension, stroke and coronary heart disease in China, Chinese Medical Journal, 92, Oct: 665-670

CHAPTER 1

NURSING MANAGEMENT DURING THE ACUTE PHASE

Introduction

The nursing management of the stroke patient is essentially one of rehabilitation. Definitions of rehabilitation contain similar concepts. Stryker (1972) for example, defining rehabilitation from the nurse's viewpoint, claims it is 'a creative process that begins with immediate preventive care in the first stage of an accident or illness. It is continued through the restorative phase of care and involves adaptation of the whole being to a new life.'

Inherent in this definition is a set of philosophical principles governing the rehabilitative process. These can be applied to any patient requiring such help, but are vital in the case of the stroke patient. They include the following:

1 The individual must be seen as a total person who has a role to play in the planning of his care, and not simply regarded as a physical, emotional or social problem. Stroke patients in acute wards, awaiting long-term care facilities, are often referred to by doctors and nurses as 'social problems'. All those involved with the patient, but especially nursing staff, must recognize the intrinsic worth of the human being, and respect the patient as a person.

2 Recognition that every human being has a right to those services that will enable him to fulfil his own greatest potential.

3   Belief that it is the responsibility of the community to ensure that the necessary services for rehabilitation are available for the individual who needs them, either in hospital or at home.

However, whatever services or human resources are made available, in the end, it is the patient who must rehabilitate himself. The most important factor is how the patient sees *his* condition affecting *his* life situation. Perceptual identification demands comprehensive physical and psychological, as well as cultural and economic, assessments with the patient and his family. Such assessments should not only concentrate on the patient's weaknesses, which are preventing his progress, but also on his strengths, which are helping him overcome his stroke. Indeed, these should be emphasized as they are central to the nurse's motivation, as well as that of the patient. The expectations that nursing staff and relatives hold for the patient will be an important influence on his subsequent behaviour.

A single, early assessment is of little value as the patterns of recovery from stroke are so variable (Nichols 1976). Rather than a single assessment a number of short, tentative assessments should be conducted in the early stages, not at random, but planned with a view to constructing a total picture as quickly as possible. The need is to identify and differentiate between short-term and long-term goals in patient care. The nurse should avoid falling into the trap of being so concerned with the short-term goals of these patients that long-term goals are forgotten, especially if the patient has been admitted to an acute hospital ward, or other accommodation seen only as temporary by those giving care (Matheney et al. 1972).

The objectives of the total nursing care plan can be summarized as follows:

1   Maintaining processes essential to life.

2   Maintaining other existing abilities.

3   Preventing further impairment or disability.

4   Restoring as much function as possible.

5   Rebuilding a constructive life.

The nurse should recognize the need to begin the rehabilitation process as quickly as possible, with realistic goal-setting and encouragement of the patient towards independence. A real danger lies in the nurse establishing episodes of meaningless activity, either mental or physical (Davidson et al. 1977).

Various aids, appliances and equipment are available to help the nurse and the family foster independence in the patient, by compensating for, or circumventing, the effects of stroke. It might be useful here to differentiate between the terms 'aids', 'appliances' and 'equipment'. Nichols and Williams (1977) define an 'aid' as a small, easily handled object which will improve a patient's functional capability. If this goal necessitates a larger, bulky or non-portable device, the word 'equipment' should be used. When the device is purposefully made for an individual it should be called an 'appliance'.

Maintaining vital bodily processes

Adequate ventilation

Position   Postural change is the simplest way by which the nurse can help the patient maintain adequate ventilation. In everyday life, if we feel unable to breathe comfortably we change our position in the chair or bed, or seek to leave a poorly ventilated atmosphere for a more refreshing one as soon as circumstances permit. The efforts we make directly reflect the degree of distress we feel. The stroke patient, because of his immobility and loss of function, has lost control of the situation.

Observation of the patient's skin colour for cyanosis may indicate inadequate gaseous exchange. Such observations are especially important in the unconscious patient. In addition, the rate and depth of the patient's respiration should be checked to ascertain any difficulty in breathing (dyspnoea). The more rapid the respiratory rate, the shallower the muscular effort, the lower will be the gaseous intake and expiration. The gaseous exchange between oxygen and carbon dioxide takes place in the alveoli of the lungs, and to reach there the oxygen must pass along the upper respiratory tract and bronchial tree. Because no useful gaseous exchange can take place along these passages, it is known as the 'dead space'. Shallow, rapid respirations mean that the new air reaching the alveoli is insufficient in quantity to meet the needs of the body tissues. Carbon dioxide levels in the blood will increase as this gas is unable to make its escape. If the level becomes too high then intracranial pressure can increase also, aggravating the damage caused by the stroke. Slow, deep, sighing respirations may not be helpful either. Carbon dioxide in slightly increased amounts can be a stimulant to respiration, excessive loss is not. If the respiratory centre in the brain suffers from an infarct, maintaining a steady, regular respiratory performance may be difficult. Poor ventilation effects a high level of anxiety, and effort to overcome the problem.

The patient's behaviour will reflect this; for example, if he is conscious, he will not sit or lie in a position which fails to alleviate his distress, despite what nursing textbooks might claim to be the correct nursing position. In most circumstances the patient will find his own most comfortable position for breathing, and the nurse should help him overcome his physical incapacity to achieve that position, however unusual it might appear to her.

The use of the back rest of the bed, pillows or foam wedges, the psychological effect of being close to an open window or near a door, or the encouragement to cough up any sputum, are simple measures that can be offered to any breathless patient, but the anticipation of the nurse is put to the test in the case of an aphasic or unconscious stroke patient.

When unconscious, the patient must never be allowed to lie on his back in case his tongue becomes an obstruction to the airway. Positioning the patient on one side will prevent this happening, but the nurse must bear in mind that this must complement the aim of preventing contractures. An artificial airway can help prevent the tongue slipping backwards. Occasionally, in hospital, endotracheal intubation may be required as a temporary measure.

In deep coma, the breathing pattern will be slow and stertorous, the paralyzed cheek puffs out with each expiration and saliva drools from the corner of the mouth of the patient, usually on the affected side. A Cheyne-Stokes respiratory cycle of apnoeic episodes may herald imminent death.

Oxygen Maintenance of a normal oxygen level, circulating throughout the tissues of the body, is vital. Without sufficient oxygen the brain cells, like any other cell in the body, will not be able to function properly at this critical time. Oxygen should be available, if and when any cell is able to use it, otherwise cell damage and the death of cells will result, and brain cells can never regenerate once lost. Oxygen should be given to the patient via a face mask, because nasal catheters are not very efficient. The Ventimask should be preferred as it allows greater control of the oxygen intake, and the looser fit is less irritating to patients. Semi-conscious patients, in particular, tend to struggle against close-fitting face masks. Oxygen therapy should only be continued as long as the medical assessment deems necessary.

Low oxygen levels, sustained over a relatively short period of time, can turn temporary cell dysfunction into permanent loss before an adequate collateral circulation becomes established.

Other methods of ventilation therapy have been studied in the hope of accelerating the recovery process. For example, the administration of 95%

oxygen with 5% carbon dioxide, or the use of dilatory drugs with hyperbaric oxygen (i.e. oxygen under pressure). However, there is no evidence as to their value in preventing the destruction of brain cells.

Adequate cardiovascular function

The nurse's role is essentially a supportive one. The medical staff will seek to alleviate any additional distress caused by cardiac dysfunction, usually by chemotherapy, e.g. diuretics, cardiac and hypotensive drugs. In cases of extreme hypertension, the blood pressure will be cautiously lowered to avert the risk of further haemorrhage. Hypertensive patients may require a relatively high blood pressure in order to ensure adequate cerebral perfusion (WHO 1971). Anticoagulants, which tend to enjoy cyclic popularity, are not usually used following haemorrhage, or when hypertension is present, because they may precipitate bleeding, and in infarction they have generally been found to have no value (Carter 1959, Marshall and Shaw 1960). Shock might be present to some degree, so an intravenous infusion and stimulants may be required, in the absence of other cardiovascular pathology. Corticosteroids are sometimes used to reduce inflammation causing cerebral oedema, but in thrombosis leading to infarction, they have failed to show benefit in some studies (Dyken and White 1956, Chandler et al. 1957). They tend to be used chiefly for transient ischaemic attacks.

The nursing care plan should take account of any cardiovascular problem or treatment. For example, all the nursing staff should be made aware of the hoped-for effects and possible side-effects of the drugs, and be told to observe the patient accordingly. Also, any activities the patient is given should be devoid of any additional stress. In the home, the nurse should explain the chemotherapy and activity regime to family members in simple terms, and encourage them to discuss their observations with her and the doctor at each visit. By doing so, any need for change either in type or amount of the drug can be recognized quickly. To discount queries with statements such as, 'This always happens with this drug', or 'Don't worry, you'll be alright', is to insult the intelligence of the enquirer. The nurse can have a direct effect in the decision-making process of drug administration. Her assessment of the ability of the stroke patient to take and retain oral medication in relation to its essential status and the need for accuracy in administration, and her patience or encouragement of perseverance in family members, could save the patient the discomfort of prolonged therapeusis via intramuscular or intravenous routes.

Adequate hydration and nutrition

The ability of stroke patients to take oral nourishment will vary between individuals. The problem will centre around the degree of damage to the swallowing reflex, or the control of the oro-pharyngeal musculature. Also important is the patient's awareness of the need for nourishment. For an unconscious patient, the decision to initiate artificial methods of feeding involves a straightforward choice. An optimistic, yet realistic, attitude should be adopted, for the longer the unconscious state persists recovery becomes less likely. The decision to commence artificial feeding should be a team decision, including the opinion of the relatives of the patient. If the vital processes of the patient are functioning normally, the decision can be postponed for up to 24 hours to obtain the relatives' point of view.

When the decision is made to feed the patient artficially, a nasogastric tube is left in situ, and a dietary plan worked out with the guidance of the dietitian. This should provide 1500 calories of carbohydrate, protein and a little fat, vitamins and minerals, and 2000 ml of fluid, each 24 hours. If no such preparatory help is available, the nurse or family should prepare a similar nutrient:fluid ratio using an accepted, combined nutrient such as Complan. All concerned should try to avoid resorting to haphazard concoctions of milk and eggs etc because, as no one can predict the period of time which artificial feeding will be required, there is a risk that any haphazard approach might cause starvation, anaemia or avitaminosis in the patient. The provision of nourishment by artificial means must always be scientific. If adequate refrigeration is available, a 24 hour supply can be made up each morning, otherwise the preparation of 'feeds' should be done separately at the appointed time. The nasogastric tube can be left in situ, providing its position is checked by a litmus-paper test prior to the nutrients being inserted. A small amount of water should be inserted to clean the tube after each feed, and any crustations from nasal secretion should be removed from the tube. The feed must never be inserted under pressure. All utensils should be washed thoroughly after each use, for although this is not a sterile procedure, it should be kept clean.

Each feed should not exceed 200-300 ml in order to avoid undue distension of the stomach. The feed should not be administered straight from the refrigerator, rather it should be allowed to warm up to room temperature, but not left as such for more than 30 minutes. All food entering the stomach sets off a gastro-colic reflex, stimulating defaecation, a fact which may be used in conjunction with aperients to prevent constipation or impaction. This reflex is most active when very cold or hot food is taken. Whenever possible, the timing of artificial feeds should coincide with the patient's usual meal times, or the provision of food on the ward, even if the patient is unconscious.

If the patient is aware of his surroundings, the continuous presence of the nasogastric tube may be distressing. The discomfort of frequent insertions related to the distress which continuous presence holds should be discussed with the patient and his relatives. All else being equal, the nurse should be prepared to acquiesce to their decision as to whether or not the tube should be left in situ or removed after each feeding, if there are no clinical contradictions. The nurse should not impose the continuous presence of the tube on the patient in order to save herself time.

If the patient is conscious and is used to wearing dentures, he should be encouraged to wear them whenever possible. Before each feed the conscious patient should attempt to take fluids orally, from a spoon and then through a straw or feeding cup. The amount of tube feed should be adjusted accordingly, until it can be discontinued. Again, the nurse must not fall into the trap of finding it easier to give the full feed each time, without encouraging the patient to try to re-establish the normal method of taking nourishment.

Throughout this period, oral hygiene should be carried out after each feed, to prevent drying of the mucus membrane, coating of the tongue, and to promote the psychological comfort of fresh breath. The action of chewing is a stimulant to saliva flow. However, if the patient is unconscious or his swallowing reflex is impaired, stimulants to increase saliva flow should be avoided. If the patient is normally hydrated, such stimulants would be unnecessary.

Intravenous feeding should only be employed as a last resort. It may be necessary however, to restore excessive fluid loss, regain electrolyte balance, or to administer a hyperosmotic solution or potent diuretic to reduce cerebral oedema. It should be discontinued as soon as the medical objective has been attained, and not maintained simply to ensure adequate hydration which can be achieved by other means. An intravenous infusion inhibits the patient's progress by interfering with his mobility. All normal precautions associated with the care of the infusion should be carried out. A flow-control meter should be used to prevent over-infusion, particularly if the patient has had a cerebral haemorrhage. The infusion should be inserted into the affected arm, and maintained there as long as possible, by splinting. Changing to the unaffected arm has serious consequences for the stroke patient.

Progressive nutritional management for stroke patients is discussed in chapter 4.

Adequate levels of elimination

Elimination includes:

1   Normal — micturition
            defaecation
            perspiration
            respiration

2   Abnormal — expectoration of sputum
               vomiting
               discharges

Discharges are not usually present in the absence of other, usually un-related, pathology, and therefore will not be discussed here. As most of the female victims of stroke are post menopausal, care of a menstruating patient does not present the same problem in hemiplegia as it does in paraplegia, so this is also excluded.

Normal   Micturition is the act of passing urine. In Western societies this is usually carried out in controlled social circumstances. Both physical and social aspects of urinary disposal are learned activities. Stroke, particularly involving the anterior cerebral arteries, can severely disrupt this learned activity, with resulting incontinence. Urinary problems in the early stages of stroke are very vexing for the patient. In the first instance, however, it is important that he passes urine adequately, even in an uncontrolled manner. Post-hemiplegic ret-ention is usually transient (Policoff 1970). The use of diuretics will increase the urine output, making control even more difficult.

The convenient strategy of indwelling, or repeated catheterization, so commonly used, is detrimental to the long-term rehabilitation of the patient by encouraging catheter dependency, which then requires an extensive bladder retraining programme for correction. Also, it interferes with progress in trans-fer, dressing and ambulation. The use of incontinence pants or pads, espec-ially for female patients who are more prone to urinary-tract infections, with frequent changes and cleaning of the perineum, is a more logical solution in the long term. For the incontinent male patient who cannot control a urinal, an external drainage sheath and tubing into a receptacle, which can be attached to the patient's leg is preferable to an indwelling catheter. Careful inspection and cleaning of the foreskin, and other areas where sores can develop, should be carried out routinely.

In hospital, such intensity of care often depends on the number of staff available. In the home, the family's physical or psychological ability to change the patient is important, as well as the amount of additional laundering incontinence imposes. The decision to catheterize should be taken more seriously than would appear to be the case, especially in hospitals.

Defaecation is not a critical factor in the immediate care of the stroke patient. Attention can usually be deferred for 48 hours or even longer. Nursing problems which might arise in this respect are discussed in chapter 5.

Perspiration is discussed under temperature control, while fluid loss through respiration is an uncontrollable variable which should be noted rather than discussed here.

Abnormal   Vomiting and nausea can be symptomatic of an increase in intracranial pressure, especially in patients with hypertension. If the patient complains of feeling sick, his blood pressure should be checked, and the presence of blurred vision or headache discovered by tactful questioning. If the patient vomits, he should be positioned in such a way as to avoid aspiration of vomit into the respiratory tract. When tube feeding a patient, unconscious or otherwise, his head and chest should be raised slightly to decrease the risk of regurgitation and aspiration.

Sputum is excessive mucous secretion in the respiratory tract. Saliva and mucous pooling in the pharynx are normally disposed of by the swallowing reflex directing it into the oesophagus, even during sleep. Sensory and functional impairment will lead to pooling, and possible aspiration into the repiratory tract, increasing the risk of infection, which in turn increases the production of more sputum. Maintaining an adequate airway, and positional change, side to side, up and down, encourages drainage of the bronchial tree. If the situation becomes more serious, physiotherapy, and in very severe cases suction, should be arranged to help remove the secretions which are preventing the patient from breathing properly. For the patient who has a chest infection, even though he may be able to swallow without difficulty, warm drinks and expectorants might help.

Temperature control

Hypothermia   Cerebral infarctions frequently occur during the night hours. The temperature of the body is usually at its lowest in the early hours of the morning, a normal circadian variation. If the patient falls unconscious on the bedroom floor, or becomes immobilized in a cold room, then he risks exaggerated heat loss, resulting in hypothermia. As the body temperature falls below 35° C (95° F), the patient will become confused and disorientated, and he will gradually lose consciousness as his temperature drops to 30°C (86°F). His temperature should be taken if his skin feels cold, in case a confusional state is caused by hypothermia and not his cerebral lesion. The usual methods of treatment should be applied, including the use of aluminium or woollen covers. Usually normal temperature is regained within 12-24 hours.

Hyperpyrexia This term means a raised temperature. In serious cases of stroke, especially when the basilar artery is involved, the temperature control mechanism, or heat-regulating centre, of the brain can become disrupted. If the patient's temperature is allowed to remain over 40°C (104°F) for a long period, life cannot be sustained. As the body attempts to lose heat, the patient will perspire excessively, resulting in exaggerated fluid and sodium loss. The temperature should be reduced by the use of loose-fitting, cotton clothing, fans, tepid sponging etc. If the body temperature continues to remain high, the patient is unlikely to survive.

Observations and recordings

Monitoring neurological changes

Neurological observations should be instigated for all stroke patients in the hours immediately following the catastrophe. How long they are continued will depend on the stability of the recordings. The size of the pupils of both eyes, i.e. the extent to which they dilate, and whether or not their responsiveness to light is sluggish, brisk or fixed, should be noted. The general responsiveness of the patient to words of command, or the stimulus of pain, should be recorded. If the patient seems aware of his surroundings, he is asked simple informational questions, such as 'What is the number (or name) of your house?' Inability to give correct answers to such questions can indicate a possible precipitation into unconsciousness in a seemingly alert patient. A reflex hammer will be required to assess the degree of central-nervous-system impairment.

Blood pressure and pulse

Blood-pressure and pulse recordings should be taken hourly, for as long as the nurse deems necessary. Increased intracranial pressure can be detected by a rise in the blood pressure with a corresponding fall in the pulse rate. The nurse ought to be alert to the fact that the body adapts to maintain normal blood pressure at all costs, and changes may not be distinctive until the situation is getting out of control. Consequently, blood-pressure recordings should not be used in isolation as a statement of the patient's condition. Hypertension may continue to be present after the stroke in some patients, while in others it is only episodic, and a spontaneous, gradual return to a lower level is not unusual (Adams 1974).

Respiration

The respiration rate of the patient should also be recorded, and it must be counted over a full minute. Descriptions of the patient's pattern of breathing should be charted alongside, for example, 'stertorous' or 'Cheyne-Stokes'. Temperature ought to be recorded 4 hourly, unless special measures are required. In cases of suspected hypothermia a low-registering thermometer should be available. The most accurate reading can be acquired by the use of a rectal thermometer, if more sophisticated methods are unavailable.

When oxygen is given, the starting time, the period of time it is to be given and the flow rate, must be charted.

Fluid

A 24 hour fluid balance recording should be started on admission to measure the patient's intake and output. Assessing the urine output of an incontinent patient is difficult. If incontinence pads are in use, the following technique is useful.

Draw up an estimate chart, by pouring measured amounts of water, e.g. 50 ml, 100 ml, 150 ml and so on, on to a pad, measuring the diameter in each instance, and allotting a figure to each measurement, e.g. 50 ml soaking 20 cm across is charted as '1'. This method of measurement attached to the fluid balance chart can provide a more accurate assessment of the patient's urinary output than 'incontinent +++', which is often seen inscribed.

Minimizing functional loss

Respiratory and circulatory stasis

Immobility and careless positioning of the paralyzed patient can lead to serious physical deterioration which may hinder his progress and, at worst, might lead to his death.

Sustained pressure against the chest wall prevents adequate expansion of the lung tissue in the lobes involved. Pressure can be similarly exacted on the lower lobes, by the abdominal organs pressing against the diaphragm, when the patient is lying in a recumbent position. The natural expansion-contraction movement of the lung tissue is essential for the interchange of air and the movement of secretions lubricating the air passages. Collections of secretions cause an obstruction to the air flow and, potentially, pathological organisms, ever present in the respiratory tract, will no longer be able to be controlled, and infection leading to pneumonia can erupt. Bronchopneumonia, which is the usual result of stasis, consists of patches of infection spread over several lobes, or even both lungs. In serious cases, atelectasis, or collapse of part of the lung, can occur, decreasing even further the ventilation capacity of the patient. The patient will develop a high temperature and rapid, shallow respirations, and expectorate large amounts of viscous, discoloured sputum. Antibiotic therapy should be commenced as soon as possible, to keep tissue damage to a minimum.

Over-infusion via the intravenous route can lead to the patient developing pulmonary oedema, which can sometimes be mistaken for static pneumonia. The patient's respiratory rate increases, but he is not usually hyperpyrexial. Copious amounts of frothy, clear or white sputum are present, making his breathing very noisy as the secretions are moved back and forth by the air flow trying to get past them. Slowing down the infusion rate and administering a diuretic can help redress the situation. The position of the patient should be altered frequently to prevent a secondary infection complicating the situation.

Various studies have shown that bedrest and his position in bed can affect the heart rate of the patient. For example, Chapman et al. (1960) claim that prolonged bedrest can lead to a progressive increase in the heart rate and the cardiac output. Coe (1954) shows that when the patient is nursed flat, rather than in a sitting position, the heart has to work 30% harder. Early mobility exercises and ambulation can decrease stress on the circulation.

As most stroke victims are in the older age groups, the degeneration of the lining of their blood vessels increases the likelihood of thrombosis developing, as bedrest continues, and the blood flow, particularly in the peripheral areas of the venous circulation, becomes sluggish. While the nurse can do nothing about the condition of the patient's blood vessels, she can do much to prevent thrombosis by instituting exercise therapy to promote circulatory flow. Sitting a patient up in bed or in a chair is not sufficient. The legs should be raised at intervals to encourage venous return from the legs into the main circulation. Exercise therapy, instituted to prevent contractures, also helps to prevent thrombosis. Pressure against the soft tissue of the calves and thighs should be avoided. The walls of veins tend to contain less elastic tissue than arteries, and are more susceptible to collapsing under pressure, interrupting the blood flow and allowing blood cell time to adhere to rough areas of the lining of the vessel. If this happens in the main veins of the leg, a deep venous thrombosis will develop, which will seriously hamper the stroke patient's chances of recovery, as rest, which is the usual treatment, may be prolonged if anticoagulants cannot be used. It is sometimes helpful to measure the circumference of both calves and thighs of a stroke patient on admission to hospital, or at home, after the stroke, because one of the first signs of a deep venous thrombosis is swelling of the limb below the obstruction. Such a measurement is also useful to assess any wasting or atrophy of muscle, which might indicate other types of neurological disorder, sometimes masked by the stroke.

Trauma

Pressure sores are areas of necrosis. They occur when external pressure over a bony prominence deprives the local tissue of its blood supply, with resulting death of tissue. Treatment of pressure sores costs the British health service well over £70 million each year (Barton 1977). The transmission effect of pressure on to bony prominences, from beds or trolleys, can be equal to 100 mm Hg. No one is immune; even healthy individuals can develop pressure sores in 6-12 hours. Stroke victims, especially those suffering from sensory impairment, are high-risk patients for pressure sores.

Careless handling of the patient can cause injury to the skin. Scratching and scraping of the skin over bony prominences as the patient is being moved must be avoided. Turning the patient, at least 2 hourly, and examining the skin for discoloration are easily instituted measures. Many devices are available to provide additional help to the nurse and family, for example ripple mattresses or sheepskins, but preventive care has to be tailored to the needs of the individual patient. Hand-rubbing over the pressure area, in the hope that it will improve the circulation, should not be practised. Rubbing can damage tissue. In one hospital study, the reduction of pressure sores in 'non-rubbed' patients over 'rubbed' patients differed by 38%, and the sacral tissue of 'rubbed' patients showed signs of tearing (Dyson 1978). Chairfast patients are more at risk than similarly disabled bedfast patients, and incontinence has been found to be an important precipatory factor (Barbenel et al. 1980).

Another form of trauma is ulceration of the cornea of the eye. The eyes of the unconscious stroke patient should be kept clean, by wiping from the inner canthus outwards, with sterile swabs dampened with warm sterile water or weak saline solution. If the surface of the eye appears at risk, the eyelids should be closed by covering them with a cotton eye pad, secured loosely by tape. Cleansing eye drops should be inserted at regular intervals.

Fractures occur easily in the elderly. When investigations, such as X-rays, are required, it is often safer to transfer the patient in the bed, rather than struggling to move him from bed to trolley, to X-ray table, and back again.

Prevention of contractures

Prevention of contractures in stroke patients should begin immediately after admission. Once the patient's condition has stabilized, usually within 48 hours, more active exercises can be instigated. Contractures are simply a disuse phenomenon, and are therefore entirely preventable. Belief that function can be restored only after some motion returns to paralyzed limbs is erroneous. A contracture is a shortening and thickening of connective tissue. Contrary to popular opinion, contractures in a patient are more the responsibility of the nurse than of the physiotherapist, because with good nursing they can be prevented, and thus the patient may never require the attention of the physiotherapist. Kelly (1966) explicitly outlined the responsibility of the nurse in terms of nurse-initiated exercise regimes for bedfast stroke patients. She claimed that, since immobility is itself a cause of deformity and thus a complicating factor with regard to patient recovery, controlled exercises would seem to be the logical preventive and therapeutic measure to be employed.

In the early stages after stroke, the two principal methods which the nurse should use in helping the patient are:

1   Proper positioning and support, to maintain correct body alignment in bed at all times.

2   Passive range-of-motion exercises, three or four times a day.

Passive range-of-motion exercise means moving a joint through its full range of motion, i.e. the extent to which it is capable of being moved without pain or undue force. It also helps the overall comfort of the patient. A healthy person changes his position in some small way every few minutes, so that having to *plan* position changes, even every 2 hours, means condemning the patient to discomfort or to resorting to his own means of attempting to shift his position, with the risk of an accident taking place (Olsen and Johnson 1967). Stroke victim McNeil (1975) claims that being unable to move for 2 hours is a long, long time, 'but, I found out, $2\frac{1}{2}$-3 hours became almost unbearable'.

Bobath (1970) claims that passive movements of a joint through its range can indicate any limitations due to obstruction by pathological changes, for example arthritis, and therefore the patient's ability to use the joint actively when he is well enough. However, she claims that, because the degree of spasticity in joints is variable from day to day and joints are used in patterns rather than in isolation, full joint range, although preventing contractures, will give the nurse no indication of future functional use, even in the absence of other pathology. Malpositioning, excessive stimulation and the encouragement of willed, voluntary effort are the three most unwanted components of any treatment plan in the early stages.

The onset of spasticity (hypertonia), which will inject resistance into the passive range-of-motion exercises, cannot be predicted with accuracy. It may begin to develop after a few days of flaccidity (hypotonia), or not until several weeks later, and can get worse for the next 18 months or so. Untreated spasticity leads to contractures.

Look at the typical picture of the untreated stroke patient! (Figure 1.1). On the affected side his leg is usually extended and not flexed. From the hip this leg seems to point outwards from the body. The foot drops down, but the toes seem to want to turn inwards (equinovarus). The affected shoulder droops, the forearm faces inwards and the fingers are slightly flexed. The patient's head and body want to lean to the affected side, and he would fall to that side if not supported.

If immediate care is not begun, this posture will become fixed when spasticity begins. The affected shoulder will become fixed lower than the unaffected one, the elbow joint flexed and the fingers fixed in a typical 'claw hand'. The patterns of spasticity in the stroke patient will bear direct relationship to the dominant reflexes. It is usually most severe in the muscle groups which flex the leg, and extend and lift the arm (Johnstone 1978). This is the result of liberation of spinal reflexes, which continue uninterrupted, accompanied by possible loss of cortical control of the higher reflexes. The normal balance between facilitatory and inhibitory nerve impulses is lost (Parry and Eales 1976a). The nurse should not assume that a patient who appears able to carry out personal-care activities soon after a stroke is not at risk from contractures, because the performance of many such activities may not demand a full range of motion. Joint pain frequently accompanies a decrease in the full range of motion, and in turn this might influence the willingness of the patient to move the joint. McNeil (1975) claims that range-of-motion exercises, 'relieved muscle ache, promoted circulation and relieved tension, more than

Figure 1.1 Typical contracture pattern in stroke

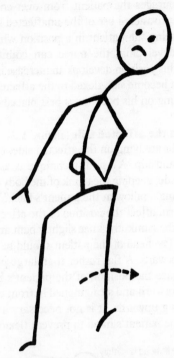

turning'. She writes, 'because my leg was so weak it rotated outward and felt as if a 200lb weight was pulling it out of its socket'. Range-of-motion exercises, passive then active, can become a morale booster and can motivate the patient for later stages when his family can be shown how to carry them out.

Splinting can help prevent deformity, especially in the wrist and fingers, but should not be used as a substitute for exercise.

Positions and exercises

It is important to ensure, in the first instance, that the bed and mattress which the patient is using afford adequate support over the entire length of his body. Boards should be placed under the mattress if the mattress is uneven. Even in these early stages, the nurse can minimize future problems by orientating the patient towards the affected side. For example, the positioning of the bed locker, television or any other objects of interest on that side, and the provision of bedpans or urinals, and conversation, as well as exercises, from the same side discourages the patient from over-compensating for his visual disturbances by protracted use of the unaffected side.

By placing the patient in a position which prevents abnormal patterns of posture developing, the nurse can counteract spasticity before it begins, because this position develops an increase in abnormal tone, and his head and trunk can become side-flexed to the affected side. If possible the patient is not nursed lying on his back; he is best placed on one side.

Lying on the affected side (Figure 1.2)   Many stroke patients find it difficult to tolerate lying on the affected side, but it is useful to prevent flexion of the arm and hip. A useful technique is as follows. Place the patient on his affected side, keeping the trunk of the body as straight as possible, and support it by placing a pillow at the patient's back. The position adopted by the trunk will, in turn, affect the position of the affected leg. This should be straight, in line with the trunk, the knee slightly bent and nothing placed under the sole of the foot. The head of the patient should be supported on one pillow and bent slightly forward. A flat rather than large pillow should be used, as the latter may displace the position of the patient's head. The affected arm should be brought forward and straightened in front of the patient, with the palm of the hand facing upwards. It is not necessary at this stage to put anything in the palm of the patient's hand to prevent flexion of the fingers.

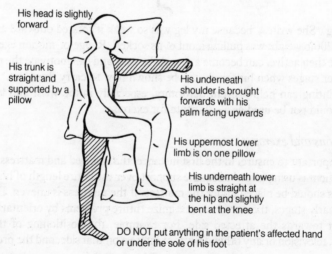

His head is slightly forward

His trunk is straight and supported by a pillow

His underneath shoulder is brought forwards with his palm facing upwards

His uppermost lower limb is on one pillow

His underneath lower limb is straight at the hip and slightly bent at the knee

DO NOT put anything in the patient's affected hand or under the sole of his foot

Figure 1.2 Lying on the affected side (shaded area)

Rolling the patient over (Figure 1.3)   Rolling promotes a sense of security, and creates awareness of the affected side. It gives the patient a better sense of normal movement than does lifting, and is less tiring for both nurse and patient. It can be desribed, in simple steps, as follows:

1   Remove all the pillows.

2   Roll the patient's hip and shoulder backwards, so he is lying on his back.

3   Turn his head to face the side he will be turning to.

4   Straighten the arm which will become the one underneath.

5   Cross his other arm over his body (both arms should now be facing in the same direction).

6   Bend his knee and place it over his other leg, in the same direction as his arms.

7   Do the same with his foot, at the same time rolling the hip forward with your other hand, so he rolls over.

8   Reposition the patient and replace the pillows.

Do not pull on the affected arm, because the shoulder is susceptible to injury, and do not encourage the patient to 'push off' with his affected foot.

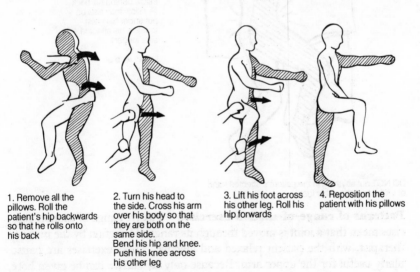

1. Remove all the pillows. Roll the patient's hip backwards so that he rolls onto his back

2. Turn his head to the side. Cross his arm over his body so that they are both on the same side. Bend his hip and knee. Push his knee across his other leg

3. Lift his foot across his other leg. Roll his hip forwards

4. Reposition the patient with his pillows

Figure 1.3 Rolling the patient over

Lying on the unaffected side (Figure 1.4)   The patient should we well over on his side, sometimes called the Sim's or unconscious position. The head of the patient should be supported on one flat pillow. The affected shoulder, now uppermost, should be pulled gently forward, the elbow of the arm slightly flexed, and the lower arm resting on a pillow. Another pillow should be supporting the patient at his back. Parry and Eales (1976b) also advocate a pillow under the patient's waist to 'stretch' the affected side. The affected, now uppermost, leg should be flexed at the knee and supported on a pillow. Again, nothing need be placed in the palm of the hand or under the sole of the foot. McNeil (1975) reported that the nusres caring for her regularly turned her from side to side, but rarely into the Sim's position, which afforded maximum relief.

Figure 1.4 Lying on the unaffected side

The patient should be fully on his side

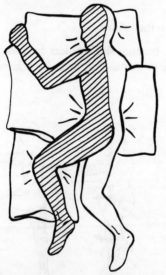

Shoulder forwards with arm on pillow

Pillow behind his back (A pillow may also be put under his waist to make his affected side longer)

Lower limb on one pillow

DO NOT put anything in the patient's affected hand or under the sole of his foot

Patterns of range-of-motion exercises   Passive range-of-motion exercises mean that a joint is moved through its range of function by the nurse or therapist, with the patient relaxed and inactive. These exercises are particularly useful for the upper arm. Because only an outline can be given here, nurses should consult more specialized books on exercise therapy or obtain demonstrations from physiotherapists.

The most important action is to maintain shoulder mobility, because this joint is the main instigator of arm movement. When moving the shoulder, the weight of the arm should be supported by the nurse placing one hand on the underside of the patient's wrist. The arm should be kept straight with the nurse's other hand supporting the elbow. All movements should be carried out slowly, without jerking and overstretching of muscles.

The three main ranges of movement are:

1 Flexion, adduction, external rotation.

2 Extension, abduction, internal rotation.

3 Flexion, abduction, external rotation.

While the emphasis for treatment of the arm is mobility, for the affected leg it is maintaining stability. Dardier (1980) suggests three simple functional exercises to achieve this:

1 Pelvic rolling. Flex both legs of the patient at the knee, and rotate the hips from side to side.

2 While the unaffected leg is left extended on the bed, the affected, flexed knee is moved from side to side, with the help of the nurse, and the patient is encouraged to try and hold the leg at different points through the movement, but not allowed to let it drop suddenly if he cannot hold the position.

3 The patient is helped to try and bridge his body, as if trying to get on to a bedpan, by drawing up his knees and pushing up his pelvis.

When the patient is able to sit up in bed but is still bedfast, maintaining correct alignment and encouraging the patient to do simple exercises should be continued.

Sitting up in bed A half-lying position, instead of sitting up, is detrimental to the patient, because the trunk of the body is increasingly flexed, and the pressure distribution increases the risk of pressure sores (Todd 1974). To achieve the correct sitting position, the nurse should:

1 Sit the patient as upright as possible, supported by pillows or foam wedges, with the head in line with the trunk and with his weight evenly distributed on both buttocks.

2 The legs should be straight and prevented from rotating outwards. Such external rotation can be prevented by a trochanter roll. The edge of a draw sheet or other suitable material, is placed under the thigh, extending down as far as the knee, then is rolled under tightly to bring and maintain the leg in a neutral position (McCartney 1974). A bed cradle could relieve the pressure of bed clothing, and a foot board might help keep the feet at right angles to the bed. Sheepskin heel protectors might be used, providing they are removed regularly for inspection of the skin.

3 The affected arm should be pulled gently forward and away from the body, and supported on two pillows.

Exercises which can be done in a sitting position include the following:

1 For shoulder movement. The patient should be encouraged to grasp the wrist of the affected arm with his 'good' hand, and raise the arm upward and forward as far as he can overhead. If a trapeze (sometimes called a monkey pole or grab chain) is placed over the head of the bed, he can be encouraged to reach for it, and attempt to grasp it with the affected hand. The primitive reflex grasp of the hand, as seen in babies, is often present.

2 For elbow movement. The patient should be placed in a sitting position, with his elbows close to the sides of his body, and with the palms of his hands together, resting on his knees. He is then encouraged to flex both arms together, lifting them until he touches his chin and then returning them to the original position.

3 To prevent contraction of the fingers. The patient should be shown how to extend each finger and the thumb of the affected hand, using the fingers of the 'good' hand. Try to get him, also, to press the palm of the affected hand down against a flat surface. A handroll, e.g. a sponge, rubber ball, rolled face cloth or other material, large enough to permit slight flexion of the fingers can be used. The thumb should be in apposition with the index finger.

Mobility is discussed further in chapter 3.

The nurse cannot ignore the importance of her role in the physical therapy of the stroke patient. Many smaller, rural hospitals have no physiotherapy services available, and the introduction of a community physiotherapist is by no means widespread. In larger urban hospitals, the physiotherapist must give priority to life-threatening situations, with the consequence that visits to stroke patients seldom last more than a few minutes. Private physiotherapy for the stroke patient at home is usually available only to those living in large conurbations, and it is beyond the means of most families to provide it for the length of time for which it might be required.

Consequently, physiotherapy services, from whatever source, need to be extensively complemented by nurses and relatives helping and encouraging the patient to adopt his own exercise regime.

Minimizing sensory loss and psycho-social deprivation

Establishing adequate levels of sensory stimulation

For the stroke patient, the need for physical intervention and care is normally apparent. However, the nurse should always have in mind the psycho-social needs of the patient, even in the acute stage of management. Sensory stimulation includes all means of communication, i.e. visual, auditory and verbal contact, as well as touch.

Even when a patient is unconscious his brain will be attempting to orientate itself to the temporal and spatial environment. The nurse can have no sure way of knowing whether touch or noise is or is not registering in the patient's consciousness at the cortical level, so she should avoid developing an approach that places a patient 'in vacuo' (Myco and McGilloway 1980). Even unconscious patients should be addressed by name and given an explanation of the procedure to be carried out on them. Conscious patients ought to be involved in discussions and consequent decision-making. This acts as a stimulus, and helps the nurse in assessing the degree of mental impairment following the patient's stroke. 'Would you like to wear your bed jacket?' demands more of the patient than, 'Let's put on your bed jacket!' which is a nurse-dominant approach.

Placing the patient in a side room or similar environment, away from the hustle and bustle of the ward or home, should be avoided. Any person kept in bed for more than a day because of illness knows how important it is to be aware what everyone else in the family is doing, to avoid feelings of isolation. Being in a side room, especially in hospital, diminishes visual stimulation. Plain painted walls afford little scope for the imagination. In the early stages after stroke, people moving to and fro provide a good visual stimulus for the patient who cannot concentrate on television, or whose reading ability is impaired. In hospital, or home, it helps to place these patients near a window, overlooking a throughway.

The need to be touched varies with age, sex and ethnic origin. Some like to feel physical contact with other people or with animal surrogates, but others avoid it. In addition, we all have contact with surfaces and substances, of many textures and temperatures, thousands of times throughout the day. However, the majority of these contacts never register on our consciousness, even though they are vital to the orientation of the brain and its ability to control the body in its environment for the welfare of the individual.

The role of the family

In the acute phase, perhaps the most important role which the family and friends of the patient can play is to provide social stimulation. However, the nurse should assess and monitor the extent to which the patient's clinical condition and general welfare is affected by each level of stimulation, and be prepared to intervene when he is showing signs of fatigue. Relatives of the patient usually feel a sense of shock in the first few days. They want to help the patient, but often feel they don't know how. Involving them in elaborate plans, e.g. exercise therapy, in the first 48 hours, will produce little in the way of results. They need to be eased into the situation to maintain their confidence, and social contact is one way this can be brought about. Sitting holding the patient's hand, combing his hair, talking to him about what is happening at home, bringing in photographs of family members and discussing them are some of the ways in which relatives can get involved. Formal visiting hours in hospital should be waived, but direction should be given as to when nursing interventions are likely and when rest periods will be in the patient's interest. Large numbers of visitors should be discouraged both in hospital and at home. Stroke patients tend to tire easily, because they cannot follow the complexities of normal adult conversation for long periods. They lose the trend of the conversation and withdraw. Rather than change to another form or level of stimulation, among large groups of visitors the temptation to talk among themselves takes over, and the patient is designated to the role that Goffman describes as that of 'non person'. The visiting situation should be consciously structured by the nurse and immediate relatives to meet the needs of the individual stroke patient.

Spiritual comfort

Spiritual comfort, although discussed as a separate factor here, is an integral part of all aspects of care. For purposes of discussion it can be divided into two categories, formal and informal.

Formal spiritual comfort   It is usual, on hospital admission, for the nurse to obtain a declaration of the patient's religion. Religions vary as to the extent of their orthodoxy and their impact on the everyday activities of the individual. In addition, individuals vary considerably in the degree to which they carry out their religious obligations, and some patients become very distressed if they feel they are failing in their responsibilities. Stroke patients are often unable to communicate the cause of their distress. Most religions allow relief from obligations during illness, and a formal communication from a minister or religious leader can usually bring consolation for both patient and relatives. As communities become more cosmopolitan, the nurse is likely to need a deeper understanding of different obligations in religion. Spiritual assessment based solely on the nurse's own beliefs is counterproductive to the patient's welfare. Statements written in examination papers about the nurse's chosen approach to the religious needs of the patient often reflect a great deal of immaturity in this area of patient need (McGilloway and Donnelly 1977).

Whenever possible, the nurse should be guided by the patient's wishes even though they conflict with her own belief. For the stroke patient in this early stage of care, the relatives may have to give directions. Most ministers or religious leaders are helpful in offering guidance as to what is essential or not, especially when conflict arises between patient and relatives. However, legal obligations, the patient's clinical condition and his level of understanding dictate the formal obligations of the patient.

Informal spiritual comfort   Informal comfort relates to the comfort offered by one individual to another, be it nurse to patient, nurse to relative, patient to patient, etc.

Most nurses recognize that certain individuals, even relative strangers, can create a more comforting effect on other people than do others. The common ingredient is usually a sense of calmness, or belief, to which other people respond. A stroke patient, who faces a long upward struggle to adapt to his condition, will rely heavily on the calmness and support of others, and the comfort they can generate by contact and example. Nurses sometimes describe this by using the word 'reassurance', though often they find it difficult to be explicit as to the meaning, and without introspection as to whether or not they are capable of giving it.

Preliminary nursing assessment

The quality of care for a stroke patient rests primarily on the nurse's ability to assess accurately the effects of the stroke in all aspects of human function. This is especially so when support from other health professionals is not readily available. Assessments are individual, but only generalizations can be discussed here.

An assessment in the early stage of care may include four critical areas, namely:

1 Extent of loss of motor power.
2 Extent of loss of sensation.
3 Extent of visual disturbance.
4 Extent of any disturbance of communication.

Other areas for evaluation, including cognitive and perceptual deficits, mental disturbance and impairment of temporal and spatial relationships will be discussed in chapter 4.

Extent of loss of motor power

In the first instance, the strength, coordination and dexterity of the *unaffected* motions to assess any obstruction to movement. A motor deficit alone should against which the *affected* side can be tested for an expected level of function. This testing should be done at regular intervals in the weeks ahead, because stroke can sometimes diminish function on the so called 'good side' of the body. The loss of motor power on the affected side of the body can be assessed by first asking the patient to make gross movements, such as lifting his arm above his head, and then by increasing the complexity of the movement demanded. For example, picking a card out of a span-like spread.

In apparently flaccid limbs, the joints are put through their range of motions to assess any obstruction to movement. A motor deficit alone should not be a real obstacle to functional recovery.

Extent of loss of sensation

Severe sensory loss occurs in only about 10-15% of strokes, but can have a profound bearing on rehabilitation (Nichols 1976). Assessing sensory loss depends on establishing some form of communication that indicates 'yes' or 'no', especially if the patient has expressive aphasia. When this happens, the words 'yes' and 'no' may become juxtaposed, i.e. he says 'yes' when he means 'no' and vice versa. These two words may be better represented by a nod of the head, a facial expression or two distinct sounds (Ornstein 1972). The validity of testing for sensory loss in a patient with receptive aphasia is questionable. Once satisfactory communication is established the nurse should proceed with testing the general area of loss of sensation, with the careful use of a pin or other pointed object. Again, tests for loss of sensation are conducted on the unaffected side first.

Extent of visual disturbance

The most common visual disturbances following stroke are hemianopia and an impairment of the patient's ability to perceive depth. Hemianopia is said to be present when the patient is unable to see part of his visual field, while looking straight ahead. The term homonymous hemianopia is used when the patient loses the nasal half of the vision of one eye and the temporal half of the vision of the other eye. For example, if the patient loses his vision in the nasal half of the right eye and the temporal half of the left eye, he will be unable to see to the right of the midline when looking straight ahead.

Before checking for visual disturbances caused by stroke, it is important to determine that the patient has had no previous deficit, such as short-sightedness. The patient is requested to look straight ahead, and then, standing in front of him, the nurse holds a pencil in each hand at the 180° limit of his peripheral vision, one pencil on each side. She keeps her arms below the level of the patient's vision in case he follows their movement rather than that of the pencils. Simultaneously moving the pencils in an arc towards the patient's midline, as he looks straight ahead, the nurse asks him to indicate when he sees each of them. The patient with hemianopia will see the pencil on the unaffected side much earlier. The defective side is tested again to confirm the deficit is present.

To test for possible disturbance in depth perception, two pencils are held at eye level, in front of the patient, but at different distances from his face. If the patient cannot tell that the pencils are not parallel some perceptual deficit may be present. Nurse learners can practise these tests on each other in the classroom.

Extent of any disturbance of communication

Some speech deficit is present in about 50% of stroke victims, and most frequently accompanies right-sided hemiplegia. Aphasia (or dysphasia) is a disturbance of language, i.e. of the spoken or written word.

Before assessing the patient's ability to communicate, the relatives are asked whether or not he had any previous problems, e.g. deafness, dyslexia or illiteracy. Aphasia can be roughly classified into three types, global aphasia, expressed aphasia and receptive aphasia.

1 Global aphasia is an inability to understand the spoken or written word, with failure to express thoughts and needs by speech or writing. This deficit can vary in degree between patients, but it affects about 15% of stroke victims. Expletives may still be expressed, and some may upset relatives and staff.

2 Expressive aphasia, sometimes called Broca's aphasia, means the patient is unable to say what he wants. It is caused by a lesion in the anterior speech cortex (Penfield 1966). Automatic speech may be present and clearly spoken, e.g. singing hymns or reciting nursery rhymes. When a patient is bilingual, he is usually aphasic in both languages, but he may retain his native language, while being aphasic in his second one.

3 Receptive aphasia, sometimes called sensory or Wernicke's aphasia, means that the patient is unable to understand the spoken language, including his own utterances, owing to a lesion in the posterior speech cortex.

The nurse can assess which type of aphasia may be present, if no other impairment, such as mental confusion, exists. The patient is asked to pick up an object, such as a pencil, from a group of everyday objects on a table or tray. The objects should be about the same size, and demand roughly the same degree of difficulty in picking up. Pointing to one of the other objects on the tray and asking the patient to identify it is a very useful test. This should be repeated several times in case the patient has made a lucky guess.

A patient may be able to understand and express himself, but have a slurring of speech owing to paralysis, or incoordination of the speech muscles. This mechanical disturbance is called dysarthria.

Although early assessment of the patient should be constructed to be systematic and reliable, intuition and imagination play an important part. As nurses we are often taught to distrust these abilities in a professional approach to nursing, but they are useful and should not be ignored. Routine responses may be practical and useful, but the nurse should be aware that once she begins to search below the surface of the individual and comes in contact with *his* vital problems, most theoretical premises can become ineffectual words, and her own creativity and imagination must be brought into the assessment situation.

References

Adams, G F (1974) Cerebrovascular Disability and the Ageing Brain, Churchill Livingstone

Barbenel, J C, Jordan, M M and Nicol, S M (1980) Major pressure sores, Health & Social Services Journal, LXXXX (4715): 1344

Barton, A A (1977) Prevention of pressure sores, Nursing Times, 145: 1593-1595

Bobath, B (1970) Adult Hemiplegia — Evaluation and Treatment, William Heinemann (Medical)

Carter, A B (1959) The immediate treatment of non-embolic hemiplegic cerebral infarction, Quarterly Journal of Medicine, 29: 611-625

Chandler, G N, Clark, A N G, Higgins, F E, Newcome, C P and Taverner, D (1957) Cortisone in the immediate treatment of cerebral apoplexy, Gerontologica, 5: 717-722

Chapman, C D (1960) Behaviour of stroke volume at rest and during exercise in human beings, Journal of Clinical Investigation, 39: 1208-1213

Coe, S W (1954) Cardiac work and the chair treatment of acute coronary thrombosis, American International Medicine, 40: 42-47

Dardier, E L (1980) The Early Stroke Patient — Positioning and Movement, Ballière Tindall

Davidson, S (1977) Nursing Care Evaluation — Concurrent and Retrospective Review Criteria, C V Mosby

Dyken, M and White, P T (1956) Evaluation of cortisone in the treatment of cerebral infarction, Journal of the American Medical Association, 162: 1531-1534

Dyson, R (1978) Bedsores — the injuries hospital staff inflict on patients, Nursing Mirror, 147: 30-32

Johnstone, M (1978) Restoration of Motor Function in the Stroke Patient — A Physiotherapist's Approach, Churchill Livingstone

Kelly, M M (1966) Exercises for the bedfast patient, American Journal of Nursing, 66: 2209-2213

McCartney, V C (1974) Rehabilitation and dignity of the stroke patient, Nursing Clinics of North America, 9 (4): 693-701

McGilloway, F A and Donnelly, L (1977) Religion and patient care — the functionalist approach, Journal of Advanced Nursing, 2 (1): 3-13

McNeil, F (1975) Stroke — nursing insights from a stroke-nurse victim, Registered Nurse, 387 Sept: 75-81

Marshall, J and Shaw, D A (1960) Anticoagulant therapy in acute cerebrovascular accidents — a controlled trial, Lancet, i: 995-998

Matheney, R V, Nolan, B T, Hogan, A E and Griffen, G J (1972) Fundamentals of Patient-centred nursing, C V Mosby

Myco, F and McGilloway, F A (1980) Care of the unconscious patient — a complementary perspective, Journal of Advanced Nursing, 5 (3): 273-284

Nichols, P J R (1976a) Rehabilitation Medicine — The Management of Physical Disabilities, Butterworths

Nichols, P J R and Williams, E (1977) Aids and appliances, in S Mattingley (Editor), Rehabilitation Today, Update Books

Olsen, E V and Johnson, B J (1967) Immobility — effects on cardiovascular function, American Journal of Nursing, 67 (4): 781-783

Ornstein, R (1972) The Psychology of the Consciousness, W H Freeman

Parry, A and Eales, C (1976a) Hemiplegia — damage to nervous pathways, Nursing Times, 72: 1640-1641

42   Nursing Care of the Hemiplegic Stroke Patient

Parry, A and Eales, C (1976b) Hemiplegia — handling the early stroke patient at home and in the ward, Nursing Times, 72: 1680-1683

Penfield, W (1966) Speech, perception and the uncommitted cortex, in J C Eccles (Editor), Brain and Conscious Experience, Springer-Verlag.

Policoff, L D (1970) Philosophy of stroke rehabilitation, Geriatrics, 25: 99-107

Stryker, R P (1972) Rehabilitative Aspects of Acute and Chronic Nursing Care, W B Saunders

Todd, J M (1974) Physiotherapy in the early stages of hemiplegia, Physiotherapy, 60 (11): 336-342

World Health Organization (1971b) Stroke — treatment, rehabilitation and prevention, WHO Chronicle, 25, Oct: 466-469

CHAPTER 2

THE REHABILITATION PHASE

Introduction

When the condition of the stroke patient has become stable, he enters into a prolonged struggle to regain his independence. He should be encouraged to do as much for himself as he is realistically able, so that he can move swiftly from a dependent to an independent state. The smoothness of this transition will depend on the preparations made in the acute phase, and the development of consistency in the appraisal of need and in the organization of care in the second phase of his rehabilitation. Consistency is an element that supports the development of confidence in the performance of a task (Matheney et al. 1972). Lack of consistency from the health-care team and family members can increase frustration and eventually lead to apathy and withdrawal in the patient. It is important to avoid the frustration of failure (Johnstone 1978).

Rehabilitation cannot be achieved without the co-operation of the patient, but his progress is often dominated by the actions of others. For example, several longitudinal studies have demonstrated that stroke victims can actually regress in terms of their functional achievements in an over-protective environment (e.g. Hyman 1972, Moskowitz et al. 1972, Isaacs 1977, Garraway et al. 1980a). Late functional improvements seem to depend heavily on the patient achieving adequate control over negative emotions such as depression, fear, despair and lack of purpose (diBenedetto 1974). In addition, patients with perceptual difficulties tend to be less motivated, on the whole, than other stroke patients, whatever the environment might be (Christopherson et al. 1974). Consequently, the management of the patient in the rehabilitative phase cannot be intuitive, rather it should be planned, as far as possible, with the patient and his relatives, so that the signs of progress can be reinforced. This demands rapport, and rapport can only be established and maintained if contacts are consistent and of sufficient length to allow confidence to develop in these relationships. Co-operation between community and hospital personnel will have to increase above normal levels, if the rehabilitative momentum of the patient is to be maintained after his discharge from hospital.

It can be anticipated that about 10% of stroke victims who survive their catastrophe will make very little, or no, recovery. Consistent assessment and realistic planning of care will help to avoid stroke patients continuing to use therapy resources either when no recovery is likely or after the optimal point of such therapy is past. Such scarce resources are frequently misused in this way (Garraway et al. 1980b). For example, a patient is more likely to receive physiotherapy if the stroke is severe, and such provision is not usually related to his condition before his stroke; his age, sex or level of mobility. Physiotherapy is often continued simply because the patient is in hospital (Brocklehurst et al. 1978).

Planning and measurement of progress demands the use of indicators of functional ability. Such indicators tend to centre on the ability of the patient to carry out activities of daily living (ADL). Activities of daily living is a phrase used to encompass all those activities an individual carries out to maintain physical integrity (Elhart et al. 1978). They will vary widely among individuals, in type and in intensity, at different times. The ADL index which the nurse chooses to use will reflect such differences, but it should conform to certain criteria in order that the plan of care can be evaluated successfully.

The criteria are as follows:

1 The index needs to be comprehensive in its coverage of activities, but also to be as short and concise as possible.

2 It should be simple enough to be carried out by any member of staff.

3 It must be suitable for assessing all degrees of impairment.

4 It should be constructed in such a way that it can be used for assessment of patients as individuals, and delineate their needs for care.

5 It must be completely objective (Nichols 1976).

A number of functional-evaluation, or ADL, indices are available which meet such criteria. Space permits only four to be mentioned here.

Kenny rehabilitation index (Schoening et al. 1965)

This is a functional evaluation form which measures numerically the self-care abilities of the patient. It consists of 18 self-care items, divided into 6 major categories, namely bed activities, transfers, locomotion, dressing, personal hygiene and feeding.

Barthel functional evaluation index (Mahoney and Barthel 1965)

This is another functional evaluation which measures the dependency-independency status of the patient, over a scale of 0-100. Areas of measurement concern mobility, dressing, personal hygiene and feeding.

The PULSES profile (Moskowitz and McCann 1957)

This is an evaluation index based on grading the patient on a scale of 1-4, in 6 categories, namely physical condition, upper and lower limb disability, sensory loss, excretory control and emotional status.

The nursing dependency index (Walton et al. 1979, Smith et al. 1977)

Developed from an earlier index by Katz et al. (1970), this form covers 20 separate areas central to the general management of the stroke patient, whether in hospital or at home. A scale of 0-4 is applied to each category. The authors claim that the form will, 'focus on the level of independence of the patient in relation to his residual disability, the level of assistance required in the performance of selective activities, and the utilisation of community resources'.

Various studies expound the value, or otherwise, of different indices (e.g. Carroll 1962, Wylie 1967 and Granger et al. 1975). For example, one study which compared the Katz, Barthel and Kenny scores of 100 patients with various medical rehabilitative requirements found that the Katz scale was the least sensitive, the Barthel intermediate and the Kenny scale the most sensitive to functional change in the patient (Donaldson et al. 1973). The value of any quantitative index rests on its sensitivity in monitoring the individual progress of a patient over weeks, months or even years. The progress of the stroke patient will tend to fluctuate, and the human memory can be an unreliable tool by which to record such progress.

The use of ADL indices can also indicate patterns of general response among stroke patients. For example, one retrospective study involving 87 patients, using the Barthel index, showed that there was no difference between the sexes in terms of the number of points gained on the scale during rehabilitation. It was also found that patients over 65 years old, although having more problems than younger ones, nevertheless made equal progress over identical periods of time. Dysphasic patients showed a greater degree of improvement on their Barthel scores than those who had normal speech, but were subject to more visual spatial difficulties (South 1971).

If an ADL index can be used as a stimulus to the early introduction of the rehabilitation process, it will help to prevent the patient suffering an 'overdose of bedrest', the results of which were dramatically described by Asher (1974). 'Look at the patient lying long in bed! What a pathetic picture he makes! The blood clotting in his veins, the lime draining from his bones, the scybala stacking up in his colon, the flesh rotting from his seat, the urine leaking from his bladder, and the spirit evaporating from his soul.'

More scientifically, a classic study by Dietrick et al. (1948) demonstrated that the physiologic aspects of immobility on the human body included a decreased basal metabolism, muscle size and blood volume, and an increase in the pulse rate, and in the excretion of nitrogen, calcium, and phosphorus. In addition, his subjects showed signs of anxiety, hostility and changes in their normal patterns of sleep and mental activity. Later authors described this state as 'de-conditioning' (Spencer et al. 1965, Kottke 1966). Loss of general muscle tone, which in a state of complete misuse can be estimated at 10-15% of strength each week, coupled with a decrease in the efficiency of peripheral neuromuscular reflexes, can lead to a corresponding inability of the cardiovascular system to adjust to an upright position (Taylor et al. 1949, Birkhead et al. 1963). In one study, after 3 weeks bedrest, even healthy young men took 5 weeks after activity was resumed to respond normally to changing to an upright position (Taylor et al. 1949).

Mental barriers to rehabilitation

As well as physical obstacles to mobilizing, mental barriers to progress may also be present. The recovering stroke patient must pass through certain milestones to progress, he must sit up, stand, walk, attain personal self-care, and eventually social reliability (Adams and Hurwitz 1963). If no straightforward physical barrier explains why a patient is not progressing, the nurse should search for a specific mental cause. The clinical picture such barriers present will vary widely from day to day. The patient is unlikely to be aware of them, so the nurse must be alert to her own observations, and those of the relatives, which might signal the existence of a mental barrier, through poor motivation in the patient. Adams and Hurwitz (1963) give a list of mental barriers to recovery, for stroke patients who have no clouding of consciousness or severe intellectual impairment, and who have adequate hearing, vision, motor and sensory function and coordination (Table 2). A few points from this list might be usefully explained here.

Table 2 A list of mental barriers to recovery (Adams and Hurwitz 1963)

Objectives		Mental barriers to recovery
Sit up	1	A defect in comprehension
	2	Neglect of the affected limb
	3	Denial of disorder
Stand up	4	Disturbance of body image
	5	'Space blindness'
	6	Apraxia
	7	Motor perseveration
Walk	8	Memory loss of immediate events
	9	'Mirror', or other synkinetic movements
Self care	10	Loss of confidence
	11	True depression
	12	Too inattentive
	13	'Don't want to do it!'
	14	Catastrophic reactions

Disturbance of body image means that the patient has lost his appreciation of the relation between different parts of his body, as well as their relationship to the space around him. Body image is a product of relevant early experience, and has its primary source in relationships and attitudes of significant people in early life. Development of a positive and realistic body image is important in the construction of a health ego, and sense of self prestige. Whether or not a stroke patient can give up his original body image and develop a compromise image will influence the success of his adjustment to disability (Trambly and Scott 1977). Patients with problems of body image may be helped by practising basic movements, such as rolling, sitting and standing, in front of full-length mirrors (Casey and Tupper 1977). Space blindness means that the patient has difficulty in appreciating the lay out of the room. Apraxia is a term used when the patient has lost the ability to initiate previously learned movements. Perseveration means a repetitive movement which the patient is making, for example brushing hair or drawing a picture, which speeds up in an uncontrolled manner, and he may be unable to stop the movement. Synkinesia relates to interference with movement. For example, when walking, when one leg moves forward the other leg may also move involuntarily. This is sometimes called a 'double gait' movement, because the patient has difficulty moving his legs alternately.

Catastrophic reactions are extreme examples of emotional lability, which erupt unexpectedly in a patient who is trying his best. If the nurse burdens the patient too much, he may burst into extreme rage, or withdraw into sullenness uncharacteristic of his usual level of motivation. The outburst is usually momentary, but it is out of all proportion to the seriousness of the task set or to the degree of failure. The nurse or family member should understand that this is a completely unconscious, impulsive action. It is not malicious or an attempt to annoy, rather it is an inability to control. Such behaviour should be treated lightly, and not become the subject of criticism. The patient's efforts should be reinforced, and his attention diverted to another activity. If the patient wishes to complete the activity interrupted by the outburst, then the nurse should help him.

As brain-damaged adults usually display a lack of initiative and appear willing to sit and vegetate, the nurse must be prepared to offer stimulation during the patient's waking hours. Stimulation is not easy to achieve in the context of a busy hospital ward. The patient needs conversation, occupational therapy or other activity which will stimulate active participation. Radio and television cannot be considered as being helpful, because they can offer only spectator stimulation, and the concentration of stroke patients is low.

In providing activity, one must be aware that the stroke patient will tend to think on a very concrete level. He is concerned with the immediate, and will tend to be self centred. For example, a cup of tea will be simply something for him to drink. He may not be capable of considering abstract concepts in relation to the cup of tea, for instance that it is made of water which comes from a reservoir, and a plant which is grown in a tropical country, dried, and so on. It may even be useless telling the patient that by adding more milk or sugar the tea may become more pleasant to drink. Rather, the milk or sugar may have to be added to the tea, for the advantage to manifest itself in the patient's thinking. One should not presuppose that the stroke patient can understand such future relationships. Having to control conversation and action at a concrete level makes for great difficulty in communication. As the patient progresses, so his ability for abstract thought may improve, and his interests begin to widen again.

As already stated, stroke patients can become very self centred. They can lose interest in what is happening at home, work, in the family and in other current events. In hospital, they can remain, apparently, totally unconcerned about the condition of other patients or the busy state of the ward. Yet they will tend to maintain, and frequently voice, a deep concern over happenings which directly affect them. This can be distressing to junior nursing staff and relatives, who can come to see the patient as selfish and very disagreeable. Alternatively, the apparent lack of concern may present itself as a sense of personal well-being, which may seem to be quite out of keeping with the situation of the patient. He may even appear euphoric at times. A skilled nurse can take advantage of this euphoric state, through establishing exercise therapy and mobility techniques before the patient becomes aware of the reality of his situation. Research has shown that people can improve their feelings about themselves, simply by thinking about their positive qualities. It is not necessary to act the role, fantasizing about how they would like to act is sufficient (Gergen 1972).

It should be stressed that changes in the behavioural pattern of the patient do not necessarily indicate that any intellectual impairment has occurred. However, it is difficult to extricate from his total behaviour the extent of intellectual damage. For example, if a patient has receptive aphasia, his behaviour will reflect that he does not know what is being said, rather than any loss of intelligence. The intellectual activities which a patient was previously capable of may not emerge for a considerable time, if ever again. He has to concentrate on directing his mental energy towards relearning those simple, physical actions which were previously taken for granted. This task is not made easier by the likelihood of a state of memory loss. Immediate memory will tend to suffer most, but the condition should get progressively better.

Mental barriers to progress can only be identified if the care process allows for continuity. The psychological problems of stroke patients receive little attention in a task-orientated nursing situation.

Stroke victim McNeill (1975) claims that she was confused in the immediate period after her catastrophe, because she had lost track of time after being taken to the hospital. As she began to comprehend that she had neurological damage, her concern turned to whether or not she would be accepted or rejected by others because of her intellectual loss. She wrote of the importance of the nurse helping to orientate the patient to time, place and present circumstances, and to give constant reassurance that the confused condition is likely to be transitory. However, such optimism must not be used endlessly if it fosters a prolonged search, by the patient, for a non-existent remedy.

Patients develop individual patterns of handling stress, and if the nurse can gain some insight into his pre-morbid personality and the meaning which the effects of the stroke hold for him as an individual, which is critical to his adjustment, then clues may be obtained as to his motivation level and subsequent behaviour patterns.

The physical management of the patient has a great deal to do with his psycho-social adjustment.

Home or hospital?

There are no clear-cut answers to questions of where best to care for the stroke patient, because many factors are involved. These include: the extent of his physical and intellectual disability; the type of home he lives in; the availability, personality and attitudes of family members; the type of hospital accommodation available, and the range of community resources in the area (Smith 1981). An additional factor may be the extent of the patient's need for medical supervision related to secondary disorders, such as hypertension.

According to Weddell and Beresford (1979), current provisions of health and social services are the product of haphazard and irregular growth, in response to the interests of health care professionals, philanthropists, social reformers and local pressure groups. Stroke victims rarely find themselves in the spotlight when demand rather than need predominates. Weddell and Beresford (1979) also claim that, 'good nursing care, the prevention of infection and contractures, and early mobilisation can be given with equal effect at home, or in any type of hospital'. In relation to community care for stroke patients, a survey carried out in Edinburgh found that dependency levels were not always the yardstick for contact with the social services. While contact with the community nurse seemed to depend on the extent of the patient's disability, assistance from the home help service, health visitor and family doctor was not (Garraway et al. 1980b). There is more likelihood of receiving services, such as physiotherapy, when admitted to hospital than when cared for at home (Brocklehurst et al. 1978).

Although stroke patients attend day hospitals and physiotherapy departments as outpatients, the hospital-based physiotherapist has little opportunity to meet with the community nurse. The concept of a domiciliary physiotherapist is relatively new, although the benefits of such a scheme have been long established (Adams et al. 1957). While providing for physiotherapy in the home, such a service should not make an independent approach to the patient, but involve all staff providing care in the community. After all, it is the community nurse who is most likely to identify the need for domiciliary physiotherapy, and co-operation between staff members can prevent an overlap of service to the patient, and increase job satisfaction through sharing the load (Frazer 1978). The community physiotherapist can also be used to teach exercise therapy techniques to community nurses. They tend to use the nurse to help, rather than instruct her in such techniques (Kratz 1978).

The type of house in which a stroke patient lives can have an important bearing on his progress. Most housing appears to have been planned on an assumption that all future occupants will be physically unrestricted at all times. There is a preponderance of housing with living rooms downstairs, and bedrooms and bathrooms upstairs. Bungalows and ground-floor flats form only a small percentage of the housing total (Small 1971). Accommodation on one level may be beneficial to a stroke victim, but rehousing is not necessarily the answer. An alien neighbourhood will be less likely to support the victim, and his elderly spouse, at a time when they are going to need it most, than more familiar surroundings.

The mobility level of the patient can determine whether he is cared for in hospital or at home. Mobility is one of the central attributes by which human beings define and express themselves. It is fairly common, especially among the lower socio-economic groups, to express performance in terms of ability to do work, household chores and shopping, leisure activities etc — performances which rely on mobility for their execution (Bauman 1961). The nurse's criteria, in such instances, may be different from those of the patient and family she is trying to advise.

Few stroke patients will be able to undergo rehabilitation in circumstances ideally tailored to their needs. Nevertheless, the rehabilitation environment demands consideration because its impact permeates through all aspects of the patient's care.

For the hospitalized stroke patient, the introduction of home visits forms an important stage in his long-term therapeutic programme. The first visit, in particular, should be carefully planned, as it will be critical to the morale of both patient and family. A home assessment should be conducted beforehand, by the occupational therapist and/or physiotherapist. It may also help if the medical social worker is brought in to give advice at an early stage. The confidence of the patient should be at its peak when the first visit takes place. Further gains in functional ability have to be measured against the patient being able to maintain an optimistic outlook, and the confidence of the relatives to manage the new situation. An early discharge from hospital, before optimal mobility is reached but while the patient is in a positive mood, may be in his long-term interest, providing the necessary outpatient and community facilities can offer the family alternative support. In one study, only 17% of stroke patients discharged from institutional to private accommodation were found to have attended day hospitals (Garraway et al. 1980a). A patient who is not emotionally prepared for separation from hospital will be more likely to put obstacles in the way of discharge. Patients should not be discharged home believing that nothing more can be done for them. A community nurse who dismisses the patient as, 'the stroke for a weekly bath', will be compounding a patient's own negative appraisal of his situation. His environment should provide for two outstanding needs, namely, the maintenance of maximum functional levels in ADL, and provision of opportunities to socialize. When stroke patients are no longer receiving physio- or occupational therapy, there is a tendency for them to become withdrawn if they are not provided with an alternative therapeutic environment by nursing staff (Hoff 1971).

Home care has an advantage over hospital care, in that it offers the patient privacy and relatively independent living, among familiar people and objects. He requires an environment where he is accepted, without hostility or resentment, where he is assured of adequate affection and attention, but without being over-protected (Hirschberg et al. 1976). Prolonged hospitalization, even with the best of motives, can lead to the patient becoming demoralized, with possible regression into a dependent state.

The progress which the patient makes may also depend on the extent to which he feels in a position to exert control over his environment. If he feels his behaviour will not elicit a desired outcome he will feel powerless and alienated. The concept of alienation refers to such feelings of meaninglessness, value isolation, estrangement and powerlessness (Auger 1976). Patients who feel powerless to make any impact tend to be reluctant to listen to the teaching and advice of staff or relatives. The patient may even behave in a manner which, at times, appears to be in direct conflict with staff, in an attempt to regain some control over his environment. Alternatively, he may become moody, submissive, withdrawn and dependent. Such reactions can be compounded by episodic loss of memory, commonly found even in the most highly motivated stroke patients, by confusion, and a tendency to emotional distress which the patient is unable to control (Roaf and Hodkinson 1977). Inconsistent behaviour from a stroke patient is one of the most difficult factors which carers have to contend with. Relatives, as well as nursing staff, are not always aware that there will be such negative attitudes to overcome, as well as positive ones to reinforce. The patient must be pushed, but not too hard (Terry et al. 1961).

All things being equal, the stroke patient is better off being cared for at home. If the correct balance of effort and support for him can be achieved and maintained, rehabilitation tends to be less strenuous, to cause less discomfort, and to proceed at a faster pace than in hospital. However, the family members who have to bear the brunt of night and day care should not be taxed into poor health themselves. They will need frequent breaks, however short, through the organization of informal relief, such as neighbours and friends, as well as more formal support from night sitters, home helps etc. Even a short period in hospital may be in the long-term interest of the patient, if it offers the relatives a rest. Feelings of guilt in both patient and relatives can do harm to a relationship, so however limited support might be, it may give a large psychological boost to the family. In helping to organize such support, the nurse should take care that the willingness of others to help does not result in further strain being added, by over-intrusion, to an already overburdened household (Whittet 1971).

The social effects of stroke on family carers have been emphasized in a study of the long-term care of 97 stroke patients (Brocklehurst et al. 1981). The results of a four-year follow up showed that the majority of survivors were still being cared for at home, but at considerable cost to the health of the chief carer, usually the victim's wife. The behaviour of the patient was reported as being the predominant short- and long-term problem for carers. They found it difficult to cope with the patient's depression, irritability, confusion and phases of being very demanding. Other stressors which were mentioned included the patient's need for constant supervision, his restlessness at night and, to a lesser extent, physical problems such as lifting, bathing and incontinence.

It would appear from such studies, that nursing staff could be more active in supporting relatives and helping them to overcome these problems. It may only need taking the time to listen. When the patient becomes completely confused and very restless, the health of the relatives must be protected and the patient admitted to hospital.

Some useful hints can be given to help to maintain the orientation of the stroke patient. They include the following:

1   Keep the patient in familiar surroundings.

2 Keep old photographs, favourite pot plant etc, in the room.

3 Keep very familiar objects in the same place.

4 Keep the clocks going, even if the patient appears to pay no attention.

5 Keep newspapers lying around, even if he shows no interest.

6 A stroke patient can often appreciate having things read to him.

7 At holiday time, it is better to leave the stroke patient at home, in the care of another relative; to move away for a family holiday can be very upsetting (Whittet 1971).

References

Adams, G F and Hurwitz, L J (1963) Mental barriers to recovery from strokes, Lancet, i: 533-537

Adams, G F, McQuitty, F M and Flint, M Y (1957) Rehabilitation of the Elderly Invalid at Home, Nuffield Provincial Hospitals Trust

Asher, R A J (1947) Dangers of going to bed, British Medical Journal 2: 967

Auger, J R (1976) Behavioural Systems and Nursing, Prentice-Hall

Bauman, B (1961) Diversities in conceptions of health and physical fitness, Journal of Health and Human Behaviour, 2: 39-46

Birkhead, N C et al. (1963) Circulatory and metabolic effects of bedrest in healthy subjects, Federation Proceedings, 22, Mar-Apr: 520 (abstract)

Brocklehurst, J C, Andrews, K, Richards, B and Laycock, P J (1978) How much physical therapy for patients with stroke? British Medical Journal, i: 1307-1310

Brocklehurst, J C, Morris, P, Andrews, K, Richards, B and Laycock, P (1981) Social effects of stroke, Social Science and Medicine, 15a: 35-39

Carroll, D (1962) The disability in hemiplegia caused by cerebrovascular accident — serial studies in 98 cases, Journal of Chronic Diseases, 15: 179-188

Casey, E B and Tupper, A D (1977) The neurologic patient, in S Mattingley (Editor), Rehabilitation Today, Update Books

Christopherson, V A, Coulter, P and Wolanin, M P (1974) Rehabilitative Nursing — Perspectives and Applications, McGraw-Hill

diBenedetto, M (1974) Optimal care for the severely impaired stroke patient, Rehabilitation, 91: Oct-Dec: 27-35

Dietrick, J, Whedon, G D and Schorr, G (1948) Effects of immobilization upon various metabolic and physiologic functions in normal man, American Journal of Medicine, 4: 3-36

Donaldson, S W, Wagner, C C and Gresham G E (1973) A unified ADL evaluation form, Archives of Physical Medicine and Rehabilitation 54: 175-180

Elhart, D, Firisch, J C, Gragg, S H and Rees, A M (1978) Scientific Principles in Nursing, C V Mosby

Frazer, F W (1978) Community physio — a new colleague for the district nurse, Nursing Mirror, 147: 58-60

Garraway, W M, Akhtar, A J, Hockey, L and Prescott, R J (1980a) Management of acute stroke in the elderly — follow up of a controlled trial, British Medical Journal 281: 827-829

Garraway, W M, Walton, M S, Akhtar, A J and Prescott, R J (1980b) The use of health and social services in the management of stroke in the community — results from a controlled trial, Age and Ageing, 10: 95-104

Gergen, K J (1972) The healthy, happy human being wears many masks, Psychology Today, 5(12): 31-35, 64, 66

Granger, C V, Greer, D S, Liset, E, Coulcombe, J and O'Brien, E (1975) Measurements of outcome of care for stroke patients, Stroke, 6(1) : 34-41

Hirschberg, C C, Lewis, L and Vaughan, P (1976) Rehabilitation, J B Lippincott

Hoff, A A (1971) Post stroke success story in the rehabilitation of hospitalized elderly patients, Medical Annals of the District of Columbia 40(10): 640-643

Hyman, M D (1972) Social psychological determinants of patient's performance in stroke rehabilitation, Archives of Physical Medicine and Rehabilitation 53: 217-226

Isaacs, B (1977) Five years experience of a stroke unit, Health Bulletin (Edinburgh), 35: 94-98

Johnstone, M (1978) Restoration of Motor Function in the Stroke Patient — A Physiotherapist's Approach, Churchill Livingstone

Katz, S, Downs, T D, Cash, H R et al. (1970) Progress in the development of ADL, Gerontologist, 10: 20-30

Kottke, F J (1966) The effects of limitation of activity upon the human body, Journal of the American Medical Association 196: 117-122

Kratz, C (1978) Care of the Long-term Sick in the Community, Churchill Livingstone

McNeil, F (1975) Stroke — nursing insights from a stroke-nurse victim, Registered Nurse, 38, Sept: 75-81

Mahoney, F I and Barthel, D W (1965) Functional evaluation — the Barthel index, Maryland State Medical Journal 14: 61-65

Matheney, R V, Nolan, B T, Hogan, A E and Griffen, G J (1972) Fundamentals of Patient-centered Nursing, C V Mosby

Moskowitz, E, Lightbody, F E H and Freitag, N S (1972) Long-term follow up of the post-stroke patient, Archives of Physical Medicine and Rehabilitation 53: 167-172

Nichols, P J R (1976) Are ADL indices of any value? British Journal of Occupational Therapy, 39:6

Roaf, R and Hodkinson, L J (1977) The paralysed patient, Blackwell Scientific Publications

Schoening, H A, Anderegg, L, Bergstrom, D, Fonda, M, Steinke, N and Ulrich, P (1965) Numerical scoring of self-care status of patients, Archives of Physical Medicine and Rehabilitation, 46: 689-697

Small, R J (1971) Rehabilitation of the stroke patient — the role of the local authority and voluntary organisations, Rehabilitation, 79, Oct: 7-12

Smith, A (1981) When home management of stroke was a success, Geriatric Medicine, May: 65-70

Smith, M E, Garraway, W H, Akhtar, A J and Andrews, C J A (1977) An assessment unit for measuring the outcome of stroke rehabilitation, Occupational Therapy, Mar: 51-53

Spencer, W A, Vallbona, C and Carter, R E (1965) Physiologic aspects of immobilisation, Archives of Physical Medicine and Rehabilitation, 46: 90

South, J R (1971) Rehabilitation of stroke patients, Rehabilitation, 79: 43-49

Taylor, H et al. (1949) Effects of bedrest on cardiovascular function and work performance, Journal of Applied Psychology, 2, Nov: 223-239

Terry, F J, Benz, G S, Mereness, D and Kleffner, F R (1961) Principles and Techniques of Rehabilitation Nursing, C V Mosby

Trambly, C A and Scott, A D (1977) Occupational Therapy and Physical Dysfunction, Williams & Wilkins

Walton, M, Hockney, L and Garraway, W M (1978) How independent are stroke patients? Nursing Mirror, 147: 56-58

Weddell, J and Beresford, S A (1979) Planning for Stroke Patients — A Four-Year Descriptive Study of Home and Hospital Care, HMSO

Whittet, M M (1971) Rehabilitation of the stroke patient — psychological aspects for patient and relative, Rehabilitation, 79: Oct: 13-15

Wylie, C M (1967) Measuring the results of rehabilitation with stroke, Public Health Report, 82: 893-898

CHAPTER 3

NURSING MANAGEMENT OF POSTURE AND MOBILITY

This chapter aims to give direction on how to assist the patient to achieve the minimal functional movement which he requires in order to carry out various abilities without excessive fatigue. The activities which will be discussed include the following:

1 Moving himself in bed.
2 Transferring from bed to chair and back again.
3 Using his hands to care for himself, for example in dressing.
4 Walking and climbing stairs.
5 Carrying out usual home activities.
6 Travelling.

People who have the normal use of their physical functions constantly perform the most intricate movements without the slightest awareness, hesitation or pain. Such persons can walk, get up, sit down, turn around, run, stand on one foot, perform different gyrations, carry objects, bend over, kick, or just plain rest. All such self-evident actions are difficult, painful or simply impossible for the hemiplegic stroke patient, because his highly integrated neuromuscular machinery has been disrupted (van Itallie 1970). The ability to conduct independent movement is important, because it provides human beings with the means to change their location in relation to the external environment. Mobility allows the individual to search for a more congenial physical, emotional or socio-cultural environment, suited to his particular needs or values. Achievement and maintenance of mobility depends on the interplay between the physical and intellectual abilities of the patient, the knowledge and skill of the nurse or others helping him, and the value which such achievement holds for all.

Hippocrates was the first known author to record the value of exercise and the stimulation of movement for a stroke patient. However, it was not until the early 1950s that physical therapy became universally accepted, and the appropriate facilities provided for stroke and other paralyzed patients (Licht 1975).

Some aspects of kinesiology (the science of movement)

A physiotherapist acquires a detailed knowledge of the mechanics of body movement during his three-year training period, and applies these principles to the therapeutic programme. One or two aspects of the mechanics of movement might be usefully considered in relation to the nursing management of the patient, because of the overlap in some areas of the caring roles of the nurse and physiotherapist.

There is a tendency amongst the public in general, and amongst nurses in particular, to think of mobility or immobility as absolutes. However, immobility is a relative term, encompassing a variety of situations in which mobility is restricted or decreased (Mitchell 1977).

Centre of gravity

The centre of gravity is important in relation to the balance and stability of the body. This is a theoretical point at the exact centre of a mass. For example, in a person who is standing still, the centre of gravity is in the pelvis, approximately at the level of the second sacral vertebra. The exact position will depend upon the age, sex, and body type of the individual (Hollis 1976). The position of the centre of gravity will alter when the person sits down, begins to walk etc. A frightened patient will tend to become increasingly rigid, and a rigid object will behave as if its entire mass is acting from its centre of gravity. Therefore, if the centre is moved suddenly, and is no longer supported by an external counterforce, the object, in this case the patient, will be likely to topple over. That is why frightened patients tend to lose their balance more easily. Interruption of the motor pathways from the cerebral cortex, as occurs in stroke, will interfere with the equilibrium reactions of the patient. These reactions constitute a series of protective reflex actions, which help to retain balance if the individual is unexpectedly pushed over (Dardier 1980). Consequently, a stroke patient who has lost the ability to react quickly to the displacement of his centre of gravity will be at risk for a fall, and even more so if he is frightened.

The nurse can provide a counterbalancing force for the patient. To do so she must pay attention to the base of support for herself and the patient when attempting to assist him. This can be done by moving the feet apart, or by using a chair of suitable height and base as a substitute support for the patient. When the patient is attempting to rise from a chair, or begins a walking movement, the widening of the base of support should be made in the direction of the anticipated movement. When supporting or lifting the patient, the nurse adds a considerable amount of his weight to her own. The centre of gravity will then be in the centre of the combined mass of both persons, so they must move as one, if balance is to be maintained.

In normal circumstances, little conscious effort is put into balancing. When carrying a heavy shopping bag or suitcase in one hand, one adjusts by leaning to the opposite side in a compensatory movement, in order to be able to walk smoothly. In stroke, the 'heaviness' in the affected side has similar consequences, and the patient will also attempt to effect a compensatory shift of body alignment. Therapeutic measures have to be introduced to prevent this occurring, and to teach the patient to keep his centre of gravity in the normal position.

Surface

All position and movement is constantly influenced by the surface which supports it (Williams and Lissner 1969). Unfamiliar or unstable supporting surfaces require control of movement on a conscious level. For example, much more attention must be payed when walking on an icy, compared with normal, road surface. Steps will shorten, and the feet will be placed down with greater care. A person taking long strides will be more likely to slip forward when his heel comes down on a slippery surface than one who takes a shorter step, as his foot comes down almost vertically. The surface also exerts control over the beginning of the walking, or 'push off' action. Friction between the foot and the ground normally supplies resistance, or counterforce, to a 'push off' movement. Lack of friction, e.g. walking on soft sand, makes standing as well as walking extremely difficult.

Inertia

Human beings have a property common to all matter, which is called inertia. This can be defined as the ability of an object to resist either being set in motion or, once moving, being slowed down. The degree of inertia which a person has is directly proportional to his body weight. For example, a nurse will expend more energy when starting or stopping a wheelchair containing an obese adult than one containing a child. Once in motion, however, the energy expenditure required to keep either in motion is comparatively small. Controlling a heavy hemiplegic limb will demand more energy from the patient, both to start it in motion and to slow it down, than an unaffected limb. The flexor muscles of the hip initiate the 'thrown movement' of walking, as the centre of gravity is placed forward. The extra energy expended will result in fatigue occurring more quickly. Muscle force is also required to stop the swinging movement of the limb, in addition to the constant supporting forces of gravity, surface friction and air resistance. Controlled deceleration is activated by the extensor muscles of the hip, in order that the heel of the foot can be placed down in the desired time and position. Loss of control over such counterbalancing forces renders smooth walking difficult for the stroke patient. He has to relearn the action of applying force, in order to initiate and direct his leg and arm movements.

Perception

Perceptual difficulties in the patient compound the problems of motor dysfunction. For example, how can the patient direct the movement of a limb, if he is unaware of its position in relation to his body? Where such difficulties are present, the nurse or therapist may have to start the required movement in the limb, and encourage the patient to maintain and then stop the action. If he cannot, the nurse will complete the movement for him.

Movement is essential for the stroke patient. Prolonged maintenance of *any* position will lead to an increased loss of the normal range of adjustments to a change of position. This will be compounded when sensory loss has occurred, because the stimulation to move at all will have been reduced.

Electromyographic feedback has been advocated as a method for re-educating muscle movement. Techniques in this area are still somewhat experimental, and they are not successful in all stroke patients. Such techniques can indicate, however, those patients who have difficulty making smooth transitions between flexion and extension movements. Electrodes are placed on the skin over the muscles to be studied, and audio-visual feedback displays the results of the effort of the patient at voluntary control, as the extent of muscle contraction (Amato et al. 1973, Brudny et al. 1976).

Finally, it can be stated that there are four qualitative aspects of immobility that can help to determine the degree of mobility present in the patient. These are: physical activity; physical restriction or limit to movement; constancy of the body in relation to gravity; and sensory deprivation to the stimulus of movement (Spenser et al. 1965).

The concept of exercise therapy

The benefits of structured exercise therapy in stroke rehabilitation have only recently been generally recognized. How such benefit occurs is by no means totally understood, as a result, perhaps, of the impossibility of isolating different elements, in order to analyze the process.

Although individual authors on paralysis and exercise can be traced in the writings from Ancient Greece and through the Middle Ages, it was not until 1854 that London physician Robert Bentley Todd began to lecture on the value of a regulated system of exercise on a paralyzed limb. He also described the typical walking pattern in hemiplegia, and for several decades this pattern was described as Todd's gait (Licht 1975). In 1890, Swiss physician Heinrich Frenkl described the rehabilitative successes of patients with chronic neurological disorders who had undertaken daily exercise sessions based on voluntary repetitive movement (Frenkl 1890). Frenkl also made the first known attempt at grading patients according to functional ability. He made four classifications: able to walk without support; requires support for walking; able to stand but not walk; and not able to stand or walk. In Paris, in 1896, the first rehabilitation centre was established, in the form of a gymnasium attached to a hospital. One of the physicians at the centre, Pierre Kouindzy, wrote the first book on rehabilitation of stroke patients. A similar centre was opened in Germany soon after, but there was no universal response to claims for the value of rehabilitation. One possible reason for this apathy could be that the technology associated with rehabilitation techniques lagged far behind other contemporary advances (Licht 1970). However, articles expounding the benefits of exercise therapy began to increase in frequency in the early years of the present century (e.g. Bucholz 1911).

The risk of an immobilized hemiplegic developing contractures was first described in 1843. Although splints and braces had been introduced around the turn of the century, there is little evidence that the medical profession paid much attention to the prevention of contractures in these patients. It was the appalling injuries received in the Second World War which acted as a catalyst to the development of theories in rehabilitation techniques. In 1945, American physician Herman Kabat evolved the idea of applying what he called proprio-receptive facilitation to the treatment of the hemiplegic (Kabat 1947, Kabat and Knott 1953).

Facilitation theory

Facilitation theory centres on the introduction of systematic exercises involving the cardinal voluntary movements of the body. By sending voluntary nerve impulses through to the brain cortex, a compensatory control can be developed, and abnormal muscle tone, which is caused by uninhibited, dominant reflexes, can be reduced. New nerve pathways can be established, and brain cells functionally related to the damaged motor cells can be strengthened. Although uncoordinated at first, purposeful association can be achieved through the patient's own will and intention. Irregular and purpose-less exercises can be counterproductive. Facilitation theory became incorporated into exercise therapy regimes in the 1950s (Fay 1954, Rood 1954 and Rood 1962). Two present day exponents are Bobath (1970) and Brunnstrom (1970).

Both these modern approaches are based on a detailed assessment of the patient's muscle patterns, rather than the movement of individual muscles or joints. A muscle which is weak in isolation may be an important component of a strong action in conjunction with other muscles. In addition, it is more usual to find a mixture of flaccidity and spasticity in muscle groups, rather than absolutes of either.

Bobath and Brunnstrom lay out treatment approaches, which attempt to help the patient to establish automatic postural reactions in muscle groups and then, gradually, the patient attempts to superimpose voluntary control. This has the effect of counteracting the primitive reflexes which are released when cortical control is lost, and which, if not controlled, will cause the typical con-tracted posture of the hemiplegic. Bobath claims it is not possible to super-impose normal patterns on abnormal ones until such patterns have been suppressed through exercise treatment. She claims that exercises which aim to strengthen individual muscles have little benefit. The patient's problem is not lack of muscle power, but his inability to direct nervous impulses to his muscles in the many varied and intricate patterns that are used by a person with an intact central nervous system (Bobath 1970).

Therefore, it would seem essential that the physiotherapist and the nurse should work in close co-operation, and with a mutual understanding of each other's role in mobilizing the stroke patient.

The main criticisms of facilitation therapy techniques centre on the failure of physical therapists to evaluate the effectiveness of their treatment methods in controlled studies. In conditions where spontaneous recovery is known to occur, evaluation of therapeutic measures is difficult. One controlled study, involving 62 stroke patients and using the Kenny index, claimed that there was no difference in the scores between the group who received facilitation exercises and a group who did not (Stern et al. 1970). Another study demonstrated that the return of function is not always consistent with motor recovery (Moskowitz et al. 1972). In contrast, a study by Fugl-Meyer et al. (1975) found that, when flaccid paralysis occurs, motor recovery follows a definable course, supporting the value of introducing facilitation therapy. They claim also that the development of contractures is not a constant companion to reduced voluntary muscle activity; 'rather, the type of care may be a determinant for the occurrence of contractures'. In other words, it is what the patient is taught to do with his voluntary muscle ability which is important, and not that it simply exists.

The majority of doctors appear content to rely upon physiotherapists and nurses to use any technique they choose for mobilizing the stroke patient. Although some techniques are likely to be better than others, doctors are not in a good position to evaluate them, and physiotherapy has not been subjected to the usual rigours of scientific criticism (Hewer 1973). One should not assume that doctors share knowledge and values with nurses about patients with stroke, in view of the socialization of both groups within acute hospitals. In a study by Kratz (1978), where the general level of expectation of care given by nurses was low, any action taken by the nurse on behalf of stroke patients was found to be satisfactory by the doctor. There are various reasons why this might be. Rehabilitation is rarely included in the curriculum of medical students, and many doctors have never visited a rehabilitation centre and are unaware of the facilities available (Casey and Tupper 1977).

Despite the contradictions voiced in an effort to understand it exercise therapy would appear to be beneficial for the affected limb if recovery is possible. The patient should be encouraged to use the affected limbs, rather than compensating by using the sound limbs, especially if some degree of anosognosia is present (Oden 1918, Adams 1971).

The environment and mobility

Surface and floor coverings

To prevent accidents, the floor surface should be flat, well supported and well maintained. This rarely constitutes a problem in modern hospital wards, but in older institutions and homes, warped, uneven floor boards, which for a normal person will cause no difficulty, may increase the anxiety of an elderly stroke victim. The majority of hospital ward floors are now covered with sheets or tiles of linoleum. For purposes of cleanliness and hygiene such covering is ideal, but excessive polishing can make the surface hazardous for a stroke patient who is attempting to walk. If polishing ward floors is necessary, a non-slip polish should be used.

Fitted carpets are fashionable in homes today. As well as helping to conserve heat in winter, they provide a smooth, uninterrupted surface on which to walk. Carpet tiles are particularly beneficial for stroke patients, because the pile tends to be short. Thick-pile carpets can present an obstacle to a heavy hemiplegic limb. Loose rugs should be fitted with a non-slip underlay, or be fastened down so that the edges cannot be kicked up. Draught excluders should be fitted to doors, rather than placing mats across the bottom of them (Rudinger 1974). Fluid spillage on tiled bathroom, kitchen, toilet or ward floors constitutes another hazard, and should be mopped up immediately.

Stairs can often assume the proportions of Everest after a stroke. The situation can be compounded if outside stairs are cracked or chipped, or indoor stairs uneven. Stair carpets should cover the whole stair surface, and be well fastened down. White markings could be placed along the edge of the top and bottom steps to outline them more clearly. Handrails or bannisters are a necessity. If possible they should be on both sides of the stairway, and should extend beyond the top and bottom stairs, to give support as the patient readjusts his balance. Handrails should not be excessively polished, because the hands of the patient will be ahead of his body and he will require a firm grip. They should be at least 1 inch in diameter, and $1\frac{1}{2}$ inches clear of the wall. If each step is too steep for the patient, half steps can be built and screwed into the stairs, in such a way that they can be removed at a later date. They should be half the depth of the step, and extend at least one third of the way along the step (Rudinger 1974). All stairways, inside and outside the home, will need to be well lit if a stroke victim is going to use them. For indoor stairways, light switches are best placed at both top and bottom.

Such suggestions are simple generalizations. Individual assessments should take into consideration the availability of a handyman to help and the cost involved.

Doors

Doors are essential to conserve heat in a room and to ensure privacy, but in doing so they constitute obstacles to stroke victims. The obstacle will be increased if the door is heavy, improperly hung or does not open smoothly and without effort.

Door handles, locks, bolts and safety chains should be fixed at a level which will not demand bending or reaching. A tray or cage, fixed to the inside of the letter box to catch the post, will also prevent the need for bending. Obstacles such as mats or furniture should be kept away from doors.

The patient should be able to close any door when he feels the need for privacy. In hospital, privacy needs can sometimes be met symbolically, yet effectively, by curtains. Nursing staff and family members should be aware that there exists a threshold beyond which social contact becomes irritating for all parties. Consequently, some provision for the patient removing himself from interaction and observation must be built into every establishment (Schwarz 1968). Doors can not only stimulate one's sense of self-integrity, they can be said to be required precisely because one has such a sense. The act of placing a door or curtain between oneself and others is a self-defining act; it conducts the message, 'I am no longer your patient — I am myself.' Violating such boundaries is violating the self-concept of the patient. The invention of the door has been described as 'a human event of significance equal to the discovery of fire' (McGinley 1959).

Furniture

Much modern furniture is constructed for its visual appeal rather than its utility value. It tends to be flimsy and unsupportive. The type of furniture available in the hospital or home can help or hinder the attempts of the patient to mobilize. As it would be unrealistic for a family to refurnish a home just because a stroke victim lives there, advice on what adjustments might be beneficial should be based on what is available. One advantage of the modern trend of periodic refurnishing is that solid, suitable items of furniture can be obtained from second-hand furniture stores for very little outlay.

Carefully positioned furniture, of suitable height, can act as a handrail, thereby encouraging the patient to walk. If he has a visual disturbance, low objects such as foot stools, pouffes or coffee tables should not be placed in his way. In a busy home, where toys and other small paraphernalia abound, it is useful to have a drawer or cupboard in each frequently used room, so that objects can be cleared easily from the patient's way. The furniture which a patient might use should be examined to see that it is the right height for him. For example, a chair should give the necessary support to the lower part of the body and spine, and allow the patient to place both feet squarely on the floor (McGilloway 1980). The furniture ought to have a broad base of support, so that it will not move away easily when pressure is placed against it.

Drawers or cupboard doors should not stick or require undue effort to open or close. Frequently used articles, such as hair brushes and combs, should not be placed on the mantelpiece, over a fireplace or where stretching or bending is demanded, until the patient can make such movements with safety.

Beds   In the bedroom or sleeping room, the bed should be placed against a wall for extra security, taking into account possible problems of hemianopia in the patient. In general, furniture should be moved about as little as possible, especially if the patient is confused. Most modern divan-style beds are very low. The lower the bed, the more effort is demanded of the patient to gain a standing position. Modern hospital beds should present no such problem, because they have a height adjustment and braking system. The hospital nurse must check, each time the patient transfers, that the height of the bed offers optimal security and assistance for him. In the home, wooden blocks could be nailed or screwed to the underpart of the bed frame, to give additional height and stability to the bed.

Adjustable cot sides are easily attached to a hospital bed, and can increase a patient's sense of security. They can also act as handrails for the patient to pull himself up into a sitting position. Unless he is confused, the patient, rather than the nurse, should decide if he wants the cot sides up or down. His safety has to be balanced against the possible diminishing of his adult integrity. A solid, broad-based, high-backed chair may serve a similar purpose at home, when pushed firmly against the bed. A 'monkey pole', sometimes called a 'trapeze' or 'grab chain', should be extended over the head of the bed. If the patient can grasp it and pull himself up the bed his sense of independence will increase.

The mattress on the bed should be firm and unsagging; otherwise, boards should be placed between the mattress and the bed frame, to ensure a supportive surface which will provide a counterforce to the patient's movement. An unsupportive mattress demands extra effort from the patient, to overcome inertia and begin movement. A well-fitting waterproof cover should be put over the mattress of an incontinent patient. Such a cover would be preferable to strips of polythene placed under a drawsheet. Polythene is inefficient in major incontinence, tends to wrinkle and makes the patient perspire more easily, thereby increasing the risk of pressure sores developing. Hospital mattresses are usually made from firm latex rubber material, and fitted with washable covers.

Bedcovers should be light, but conserve body heat. Stroke patients are often elderly, and their immobilization increases the risk of hypothermia. A suitable degree of warmth is a premium factor, even in summertime. Nylon materials might be easily washed and dried, but they tend to make the patient feel hot, and make him slip down the bed more readily. Continental quilts are light, and conserve heat efficiently but still allow leg movement. Elderly patients, however, tend to prefer more traditional coverings, so cellular blankets are useful alternatives. In the early stages of rehabilitation, a bed cradle, which fastens under the mattress, will allow freedom for leg movement, and this encourages the patient to practise his leg exercises.

At least five pillows should be available to give the patient support. Feathers are preferred to latex rubber as a filling, even if somewhat more expensive. This is because such a filling allows the pillow to be shaped or flattened more easily, for use in different forms of support. Protective, waterproof coverings should be put on one or two of the patient's pillows, particularly if the patient is perspiring excessively.

A commode is a vital piece of furniture in the early stages of rehabilitation. They can usually be obtained on loan, for use in the home, from the local social services department.

Sheepskins   Medical sheepskins are an invaluable aid in the prevention of pressure sores, as well as increasing the general comfort of the bedfast or chairfast patient. They can be obtained from most social services departments. The wool fibres of the sheepskin distribute the weight of the patient over a wide area, and the pile helps air to circulate more freely. This has the effect of reducing the tendency to produce localized pressure points on the patient's skin, and helping to keep the skin dry. In addition, each sheepskin will absorb up to a third of its weight in fluid, before it begins to feel moist (Nichols 1971). The leather backing helps to prevent the patient slipping down the bed, but does not interfere with the washing of the sheepskin, by hand or machine. When the patient attempts to move to the side of the bed, prior to transfer, the sheepskin fibres provide a smooth, nonabrasive surface against which the patient's skin can move.

Nichols (1971) recommends the following cleansing instructions, which can be given to the relatives of the patient:

1   The sheepskin should be changed every 7 days if it is in general use, every 5 days for a heavily perspiring patient and every 2-3 days if the patient has an open pressure sore.

2   If the sheepskin is soiled, it should be sponged thoroughly with cold water.

3   Gentle handwashing, in warm, not hot, water, using normal domestic washing powder, should prove satisfactory. Alternatively, 10 minutes' gentle agitation in a washing machine will also clean the skin.

4   Rinsing should be done with fresh water.

5   The sheepskin should be hung out to dry, if possible in the open air. It should not be placed close to a radiator, as this will harden and spoil the skin.

6   The wool fibre can be restored by combing the pile with a wire brush.

Whenever possible, bedside lockers or tables should be of a suitable height, so that the patient does not risk overbalancing when reaching out to them. An additional top might be fitted on to a low table at home, raising the main surface for use by the patient, while providing a shelf under which objects might be stored. The locker or table should normally be placed on the unaffected side of the patient. When it is considered necessary to make the patient more aware of his affected side, his locker should be placed on that side, to offer an incentive for him to turn in that direction. A bed table, especially one which will fit across the bed and can be adjusted for height, is a useful acquisition for home management. Alternatively, if a patient has to have his meals in bed, a tray fitted with legs will give more support than one which balances on his knees.

Electrical appliances

Most modern-style homes are heavily reliant upon a variety of electrical appliances to maintain various functions, e.g. cooking. This is so much so that the action of switching off and on, pushing in plugs etc, is taken for granted. Simple though this may be for the able-bodied, it can offer a serious challenge to all elderly disabled, including stroke victims, not the least reason being that many electrical points are sited close to the floor.

The safety, or otherwise, of electrical appliances should be included in any home assessment by the occupational therapist. Nevertheless, the community nurse should be alert to any electrical or other energy hazard during her routine visits. Electrical underblankets can be a particular danger. They should never be used for an incontinent patient, or one who might upset a bedpan or urinal. They should always be switched off before the patient gets into bed. An electric overblanket, switched to a low thermostatic control for night use, might be safer. Hot water bottles should also be removed before the patient gets into bed, or before an electric over or under blanket is switched on.

The relatives of the patient can receive advice from their local electricity or gas officials regarding the safe use of appliances. Leaflets are usually available from local showrooms. For example, the electricity services' booklet, *Making Life Easier for Disabled People*, is available free of charge.

Hoists

The value or otherwise of using a hoist in order to move a stroke patient is what concerns us here, rather than the types of hoist available, which have been described in detail by other authors (e.g. Tarling 1980).

In hospital wards, hoists are usually available, but are not generally utilized by nursing staff when attempting to move patients. Nurses tend to prefer more traditional methods of lifting, often placing themselves and the patient at risk. The purchase of a hoist for a particular hospital ward requires careful consideration. Too frequently, the same model of hoist tends to be purchased for all wards, regardless of the need to meet the transfer requirements of different patient groups. Nursing staff must insist that they are always consulted before such equipment is chosen. The purchase of equipment such as hoists, that lies unused, is a waste of scarce resources.

A hoist can be of great value when a stroke patient is severely disabled by flaccid or spastic dysfunction or by obesity, or when nursing help is in short supply. The efficient use of the hoist, however, depends upon adequate training and practice. Such training helps to instil the necessary confidence, in both nurse and patient, as to the reliability of the hoist. Adequate tuition usually results in their being used by staff. Nurse training schools claim that they teach learners the correct situations and methods for using hoists. A survey carried out by the Disabled Living Foundation, in 1978, in conjunction with the Royal College of Nursing, reported that, while the majority of schools of nursing taught the basic theory of lifting, and using hoists, only 30% stated that they provided post-basic training in their use. The majority used only one model of hoist in their demonstrations. In the same survey, it was reported that only a small number of social service departments lay down guidelines for the provision of hoists to families (Tarling 1980).

However willing staff or relatives may be to use a hoist, especially when bathing patients, the construction of bathrooms in older hospitals and in modern homes often prevents their being utilized. Additionally, modern baths tend to be set low, and are often boxed in, thereby preventing the base of the hoist fitting under the bath. Other considerations when providing a hoist for home use include whether or not the carer can move the hoist around, the availability of storage space when the hoist is not in use, and the degree of interference it might cause for other family members.

There are two main models of mechanically operated hoist currently available. One has a fixed seat, usually made of heavy-duty plastic. This type is strong, but somewhat inflexible, and may not be suitable for use in the home. The sling variety of hoist comes with many variations. Those with only two slings should not be used for severely flaccid patients, unless the appendages can be secured together to avoid the risk of the patient slipping down between the two slings. The harness type of sling offers more support, and some have a toilet aperture in the material. Slings are available in nylon material, which can easily be washed and dried.

In the bathroom, metal handrails may be more useful than a hoist, if the patient has some mobility. They should be fitted to the wall by the lavatory, on the side of the bathtub if possible, or on to the wall just above the rim of the bath. The exact placement and height of the rails will depend on the individual requirements of the patient. Disabled persons generally need more room to manoeuvre than the able bodied, so any unnecessary objects should be cleared away, especially in the bathroom.

The requirement of complete privacy for personal hygiene is only a recent phenomenon. Modern bathrooms are constructed, in size and design, to emphasize that such activities should be performed in private and alone. Consequently, families tend to have what might be construed as a morning bathroom ritual. This usually involves unwritten regulations as to who goes first, how long they may take etc (Kira 1967). The hygiene requirements of the stroke patient may be very time consuming, and may have to be organized so as to comply with any such family arrangements.

When using the bath, the patient may find that shallow wood steps pushed up against the side of the bath help him get in and out. A bath seat and a nonslip bath mat may help him to maintain his confidence in his ability to transfer.

The lavatory seat for the stroke patient should be approximately the same height as the bed. Plastic raised seats which clip on to the lavatory bowl can be obtained. Alternatively, a raised seat attached to a frame, and which fits over the whole pedestal, might be preferred, so that other family members can remove it when they wish to use the lavatory.

The main objective in assessing the environment of the patient in relation to mobility, should be to ensure his safety, and that of his helpers. The second objective should be to arrange the environment to maximize his freedom of movement, by removing obstacles and installing appropriate aids and equipment. While the prescribing of aids to daily living and providing adaptations to the home of the patient may have an important bearing on the outcome of stroke rehabilitation, patients may derive no benefit if their 'accessory' aids, such as spectacles, hearing aids and dentures, are not in working order (Garraway et al. 1980).

Transferring the patient from bed to chair

The decision about when to begin to transfer the patient out of bed, and into a chair, demands careful consideration by nursing staff. If there are no clinical contraindications, a schedule should be drawn up, with the help of the physiotherapist, for staging the learning of the transfer technique by the patient. Each stage or movement should have adequate periods of rest built into it. (Figure 3.1)

The patient should gradually become accustomed to the upright position and develop sitting balance before transfers are attempted (Rantz and Courtial 1978). Planning is vital, as the stroke patient will not be enthusiastic about the prospects of getting up in a chair if, despite his protests, he is continually left in the chair until he is fatigued.

Conventional nursing wisdom dictates that, in organizing nursing care for ill patients, many procedures are done together, and then the patient is allowed to rest. However, Mitchell et al. (1981) measured a cumulative increase in intracranial pressure in patients, related to simple activities such as turning the body, passive range-of-motion exercises and head rotation, even when such activities were spaced 15 minutes apart. No such cumulative increase was found with activities spaced at least 1 hour apart. They concluded that performing closely spaced activities on patients with intracranial hypertension may increase the pressure further, and put the patient at risk.

Figure 3.1 Getting out of bed

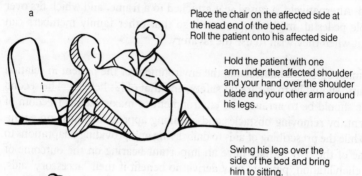

Place the chair on the affected side at the head end of the bed.
Roll the patient onto his affected side

Hold the patient with one arm under the affected shoulder and your hand over the shoulder blade and your other arm around his legs.

Swing his legs over the side of the bed and bring him to sitting.

Rearrange clothes, etc.

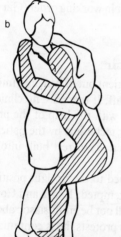

Rock or wriggle him to the edge of the bed. Place your hands over his shoulder blades with his arms resting on yours.
He must not grip his hands together or he will pull your neck.
Make sure both of his feet are flat on the floor, KEEP YOUR BACK STRAIGHT! And bend your knees. Wedge his feet and knees with yours.

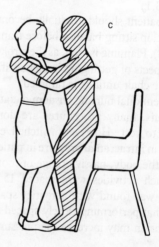

Bring both of his shoulders well forwards to get his body weight over both feet.
DO NOT LIFT HIM.
Use your weight to counterbalance his by pressing downwards and forwards on his shoulders and leaning slightly backwards to bring him up to standing.
With his shoulders fixed by your hands and his knees fixed by yours pivot him round, keep his shoulders forward and lower him down into the chair.

Therefore, patients whose stroke is the result of hypertension and cerebral haemorrhage will require their ambulation schedule to be arranged so as to give long periods of rest between activities.

Lack of rest and frustration go hand in hand. Nevertheless, too much rest can lead to a lack of initiative in the patient. Estimating the correct levels of rest and activity required by an individual patient demands a high degree of skilled observation from the nurse. She should begin such an assessment by planning short periods of activity for the patient, and note any apparent tiredness or tendency to frustration. The patient's need for rest will decrease in time, even in hospital. Frustration can be damaging, because it arises out of an inability to react satisfactorily to stimulation, and leads in time to a turning away from the task in hand, the development of an emotional reaction and, at times, 'catastrophic behaviour'.

Considerations which will have to be taken into account when planning a mobility schedule for the stroke patient can be summarized as follows:

1 His overall physical condition.

2 The degree of mobility which he has achieved.

3 His physical strength.

4 His sense of balance.

5 His level of comprehension.

6 His motivation (Stryker 1972).

The weight of the patient can be a critical, physical factor in immobility. If the patient is more than 10% over expected body weight, then a reduction diet must begin immediately. Extremely obese stroke patients have little hope of survival unless they can be mobilized early, because for all patients loss of muscle strength and atrophy can begin after only 3 days of bedrest.

Rehabilitation is often limited to the means which will enable the most to be made of spontaneous recovery. Optimism, encouragement and constant reassurance are sometimes the most important ingredients of the early mobilization phase. There is usually more hope of recovery in the leg than in the arm, especially if the patient can lift an extended leg off the bed in 2 or 3 weeks, and dorsiflex the foot within 4-6 weeks, of the onset of stroke (Hurwitz and Adams 1972). The ability to stand and walk involves more primitive acquisitions than the precision actions of the hand and arm, so balancing, standing and walking exercises can stimulate a positive supporting response in the stroke patient.

As soon as the patient can tolerate an upright position for 10 minutes, it is safe to begin transfer training. Just sitting on the edge of the bed, dangling his legs, gives him an opportunity to start developing his sense of sitting balance. This is essential for when he begins to dress himself, and is good preparation for developing standing balance for walking (Anderson 1970). Once he has learned the ability to pivot-transfer into a chair, he can extend this technique to similar types of transfer, e.g. from a chair to a commode, or from a wheelchair to a lavatory seat, and back again. In addition, once he is able to tolerate chair sitting, the patient can assist in the performance of personal hygiene activities.

This must take place with the patient's understanding and co-operation. It can be a very frightening time for him if he is suddenly transferred into a chair, without any explanation or the chance to move himself. Manhandling a stroke patient out of bed can damage his shoulder joint, as well as putting at risk the back of the nurse or relative. It is far easier if the nurse learns to utilize the normal patterns of movement, which we all use when getting out of bed every morning.

These patterns of movement can be expressed as a series of stages, designed to place emphasis on the hemiplegic side and to encourage weight-bearing on the affected limb. These stages of transfer are as follows:

1 Place the chair parallel to the head of the bed, on the patient's affected side. This will allow the nurse to work from in front of the patient.

2 Roll the patient onto his affected side using the method described on page 31.

3 The nurse places one arm under the patient's affected shoulder, so that her hand is positioned over the shoulder blade on that side. She then places her other arm around the legs.

4 Swing the legs of the patient over the edge of the bed, and bring him into a sitting position. Patients are commonly taught to lift the affected limb with the unaffected one. While this encourages independence, it may be harmful in the long term, because it produces asymmetry in body alignment.

5 Rearrangement of his clothing may be necessary, because the sitting activity elongates the trunk and clothing becomes displaced. If a pause is required to adjust clothing, or an in-dwelling catheter, the patient can prop himself on the affected elbow, taking the weight through the arm.

6   Rock or wriggle him towards the edge of the bed.

7   The nurse stands in front of the patient, placing her arms under his shoulders, with her hands over his shoulder blades, and with the hands of the patient over her shoulders. The patient should not be allowed to grip his hands behind the nurse's neck, or there will be a risk of injury.

8   The nurse should check that both the patient's feet are flat on the floor.

9   Keeping her back straight, the nurse will bend her knees, wedging or blocking the patient's feet and both his knees with her own. This prevents his feet slipping forward, and stops the affected knee from buckling under, when he stands. Both the patient and nurse should be wearing firmly fitting shoes or other footwear. The patient should never be transferred wearing only stockings or socks, even on non-slip floors (Waddington and Hollis 1980).

10   Bring both the patient's shoulders well forward to get his body weight over his feet. He should be told to keep his head bent forward whenever he attempts to stand or sit down. If left to himself, a stroke patient tends to stand up by thrusting backwards into total extension, and therefore has to pull himself forward and upwards with his unaffected arm. This is neither safe, nor therapeutically desirable.

The nurse uses her weight to counterbalance that of the patient, by leaning slightly backwards, to bring him up to a standing position. It is important that both nurse and patient move together as one. The patient must not be lifted.

Preparatory to standing, the patient can increase his confidence by practising lifting his bottom a few inches off the bed at a time, and then placing himself to the left or right of his original position.

11   With his shoulders still supported by the nurse's hands, and his knees wedged against hers, the patient is pivoted round. He should be told to pivot on his toes, swinging the heel in the direction of the movement. Keeping his shoulders and head well forward, lower him into the chair. He should not put a hand on the chair behind him, as this spoils the symmetry of the movement, and may cause him to lose his balance. It is usually easier for the patient to transfer to the unaffected side, until he gains confidence.

12   Finally, his clothing should be readjusted as necessary (Todd 1974, Parry and Eales 1976).

When sitting in a chair, the patient should sit well back, and not slouch. Padding the chair with pillows should not be necessary if the chair bottom gives support to the thighs, and has a high back, which can give support up to the level of his shoulder blades. His head and trunk should be in line with each other, and his affected upper arm should be forward at the shoulder and supported on a pillow, on a table. Both feet should be flat on the floor, so that the patient's hips, knees and ankles are at right angles. This will help to ensure that his body weight is evenly distributed over both buttocks.

If the patient has a tendency to fall to the affected side when sitting, he can be trained to regain his balance. The nurse places one hand on each shoulder of the patient, and applies gentle pressure on alternate sides, while telling the patient to resist the pressure. Once resistance is felt, the pressure is released. The patient should be sitting correctly, and evenly balanced again, before the exercise is repeated (Figure 3.2).

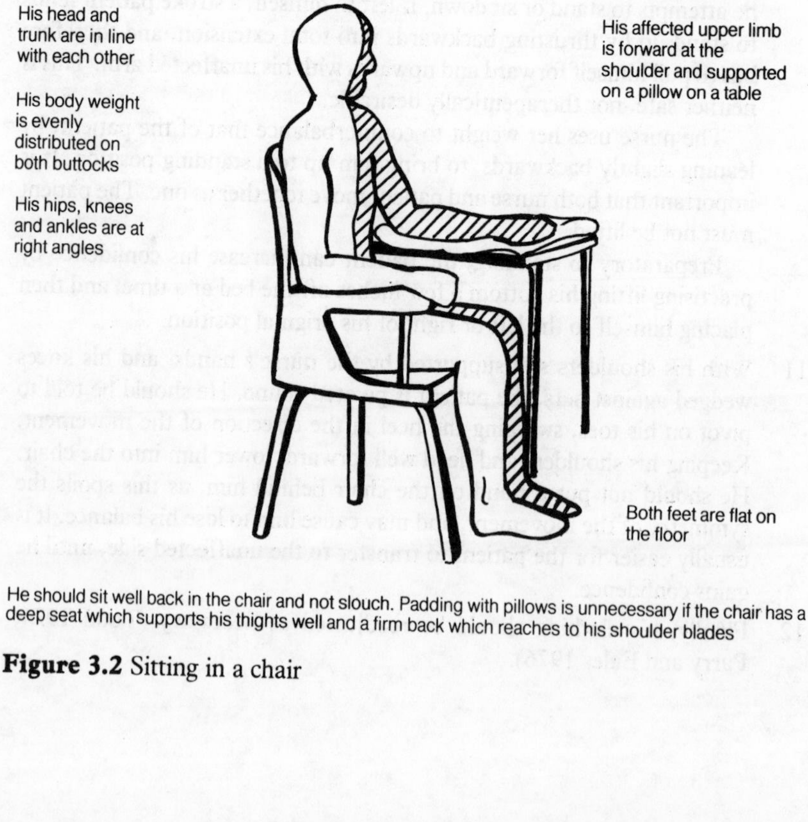

His head and trunk are in line with each other

His body weight is evenly distributed on both buttocks

His hips, knees and ankles are at right angles

His affected upper limb is forward at the shoulder and supported on a pillow on a table

Both feet are flat on the floor

He should sit well back in the chair and not slouch. Padding with pillows is unnecessary if the chair has a deep seat which supports his thights well and a firm back which reaches to his shoulder blades

Figure 3.2 Sitting in a chair

Standing

Standing and balancing exercises should utilize parallel bars whenever possible or, alternatively, two high-backed and broad-based chairs. The patient should practise stand-up exercises at least six times each day, and each cycle should be repeated about ten times, at a rate of about 2/min (McNeil 1975). Sitting up in a chair can become unbearable if the patient cannot relieve the pressure on his ischial prominences, from his gluteal muscles and the chair surface. Ideally, he should stand up at half-hourly intervals. As well as preventing undue pressure, the resulting flexion and extension of the hip and knee joints represent good therapy for him between programmed sessions of physiotherapy. In addition, stand-up exercises will help to tone his leg and back muscles.

The patient can be taught to do an exercise, often called 'bed ending', by himself. The patient sits on a chair facing the end of a high bed, with his toes pressed against a board to stop his feet slipping forward. He holds on to the rail of the bed and pulls himself into a standing position, and then gently lowers himself back into the chair, while keeping his weight evenly balanced over both legs. This should be done just once or twice to begin with, and then gradually increased until the patient gains confidence in his ability to stand (Jones 1974). As soon as possible, however, he should adapt to the 'push up' method of getting up from a chair.

Once the patient reaches a standing position, he must be encouraged to adopt the most stable position he can. In this position, he cannot be allowed to balance by pushing or pulling with his unaffected hand, because such an action will prevent the re-education of normal balance and righting reactions throughout the body.

The position of the head dominates the posture of the rest of the body, so he must be reminded to try to keep his head in the midline, by looking straight ahead, with his chin well up. By doing this, his spinal column and shoulder girdle will stay in their correct position, and his weight will be spread more evenly over his lower limbs. When standing, a stroke patient will tend to place his weight on the affected side, with the result that his pelvis tilts in that direction. If the affected leg is carefully placed, with particular attention to the ankle and foot, it will help to overcome this tendency.

About 30% of stroke patients develop an ankle contracture because they have a tendency to stand with the affected heel off the ground, and with the ball of the foot in contact with the floor (Policoff 1970, Stryker 1972). This is known as plantar flexion. The patient will not be able to walk normally if he cannot be taught to place the whole foot on the ground and place his weight upon it. By placing the foot correctly on the ground, there will be a reinforcement of the underlying mechanism as weight is placed upon it, and the patient may be able to stand. If he has adopted the desired posture, his hip on the affected side will be pushed well forward. Good hip control is necessary in order to prevent the affected knee locking in hyperextension, sometimes called 'back knee' deformity. If the hip is kept forward, the knee will not lock (Todd 1974). Back-knee deformity occurs in patients who have some degree of voluntary function. It results from a strong quadriceps muscle combined with hamstring weakness. The weak posterior leg muscles cause the associated ligaments to stretch, so that the knee locks in hyperextension. Lack of knee control makes for an unstable gait, which is particularly noticeable when the patient climbs stairs. To overcome it, he should be encouraged to bend his affected knee slightly, and learn to climb stairs leading with the affected leg. A leg brace might be needed to reverse this deformity (Hirschberg et al. 1976). A tripod or other type of walking appliance should not be used by the patient because it encourages an abnormal stance. Reliance on a tripod or cane means that the unaffected hand will be occupied, and therefore unavailable for other things, such as re-arranging clothing for toilet purposes, carrying objects etc.

When a patient learns to stand up from a chair with arms, the nurse should first check to see if he is sitting correctly, i.e. with his back straight, chin up and head in midline. His hips should be level, and feet placed flat on the floor and sufficiently apart to broaden the base of support. Then, holding a chair arm with each hand, he is asked to place his head and body weight forward. He should then be instructed to push down on the chair arms, keeping his own arms close to his sides, to prevent shoulder strain. If two nurses are helping a patient to stand up from an armchair, they must not attempt to lift him up by his shoulders, grasping his wrists so his elbows are flexed, with the result that he is hanging, or suspended, between them. Rather, they should place their hands at the level of the chair arms, so that the patient can push down on them, while the nurse's other hands support his elbow joints. As he stands up he must avoid rotating his pelvis, skewing around in the chair and trying to lift up by placing weight only on the unaffected side. He should stand up with both halves of his body level.

When sitting down into the same style of chair, it should be placed so it just touches the back of the patient's legs. He should then be asked to bend forward from his hips, again keeping both halves of his body moving together, and take hold of the arms of the chair. The patient then transfers his weight to his hands, and keeping this weight over his feet and his shoulders well forward, he lowers himself into the chair, and then readopts the correct sitting posture. When he is sitting, the fingers of the affected hand should not be overflexed, and the thumb should be in apposition with the index or first finger. Any flexion deformity of the wrist can be corrected with a light plastic splint, which can be removed during therapy.

Balancing practice can be conducted while the patient is standing. The shoulder pressure movement described on page 76 can be used. The patient should be standing between parallel bars, or other support, when this exercise is carried out.

Subluxation of the shoulder joint

More than 50% of stroke patients develop some degree of shoulder pain in the hemiplegic arm (Stryker 1972, Hirschberg et al. 1976). The weight of the affected arm alone may cause injury to the shoulder joint by stretching the ligaments (Chuco 1971). Careless handling, especially pulling on the arm when bathing, turning, dressing or transferring the patient, will cause such damage. When there is sensory loss as well as functional disability, the patient may not report any injury, and it is unlikely he would notice until he begins to sit up anyway. The hemiplegic arm should be supported when the patient is in an upright position, possibly by a properly applied sling (Figure 3.3). When

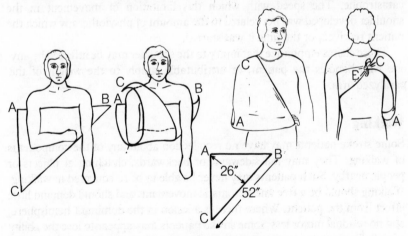

Figure 3.3 Application of a sling to the affected arm

standing or walking, wearing a sling can help the patient to maintain his balance, because it supports the heaviness of the arm (McCartney 1974). Wearing a sling will also help to prevent oedema of the fingers and hands. The sling should only be used in the flaccid stage, and should be discarded when there is evidence of recovery of function, or sufficient spasticity to prevent a diastasis of the shoulder joint (Moskowitz 1969). Then a large pillow can be used to give the arm and joint support when the patient is sitting up. The nurse or relative should keep reminding the patient to keep the affected shoulder well forward. Not all authors approve the use of slings, some claiming that they do not appose the joint surfaces adequately, and that they tend to hold the arm in a position of dominant spasticity (e.g. Dardier 1980). However, slings appear to have general approval, providing that they are removed regularly and the joint exercised.

Subluxation can often occur as a delayed painful complication. It may respond to the application of heat to the shoulder joint, with persistent range-of-motion exercises commensurate with the patient's tolerance of pain. Application of cold may also relieve the pain. Success can be said to have been achieved when the patient can move his affected arm upward, directly over his head (Kurasik and Sutton 1969).

Brocklehurst et al. (1978) claimed that, in a study of 135 stroke patients, stiff and painful shoulders were present in 21 patients by 2 weeks after the onset of stroke, and had developed in a further 37 patients by 1 year after their catastrophe. The speed with which this limitation of movement in the shoulder developed was not related to the amount of phsyiotherapy which the patient received, or the time it was started.

These claims emphasize that injury to the shoulder may be inflicted by anyone who handles the patient, or attributable simply to the weight of the paralyzed arm.

Walking

Some stroke patients may have no recollection about any of the components of walking. They may fall sideways, or backwards, clutching at objects or people nearby. Such patients may never be able to be re-educated in walking. Walking should be a free and automatic movement, and should demand little effort from the patient. Where there is a lesion in the dominant hemisphere, and no residual motor loss, some stroke patients may appear to lose the ability to walk for no apparent reason. 'After a few steps the patient feels he can go no further, but with coaxing, and by dint of concentration upon the movement of the legs, the patient can start again' (Critchley 1931). This phenomenon is know as Pétren's gait.

Careful consideration will have to be given to the point where the patient will be asked to begin to walk. It should not be attempted without proper support for the weak foot. After 1-2 weeks of standing exercises, the majority of stroke patients will be able to support their weight on the affected leg (Hirschberg 1958). Walking, even on a level surface, should not be attempted before stand-up exercises have been introduced.

To walk normally the patient will have to be able to bend his foot, lift the unaffected leg off the ground and support his weight, momentarily, on the affected limb. If he cannot bend his foot, and drags his toes when walking, a plastic brace or caliper which is light but sturdy may be prescribed. Because of the psychological trauma which bracing may effect, any decision to prescribe a permanent brace should be postponed for 6-12 weeks after the onset of stroke (Policoff 1970).

Most leg braces fit below the knee and have an ankle piece, shaped like a stirrup and with a posterior strap, fitted to prevent flexion when the foot is lifted up. Some authors mention the inclusion of a toe spring, fitted to the brace, to keep the toes from dropping. However, toe springs should not be used where there is excessive spasticity with clonus. Clonus is alternate contracture and relaxation of muscles, in rapid succession, due to CNS damage. It occurs particularly in the ankles and wrists, and can be triggered off by a sudden change in position. Long leg braces are rarely used, because they tend to be heavy and clumsy, and interfere with activities such as dressing. They may be prescribed, however, for stroke patients with particular problems, for example a persistent back-knee deformity.

If deformity prevents the patient walking, surgical intervention may become necessary. For a foot inverted inwards, half of the tibialis anterior muscle may be transplanted to the outer side of the foot. For equinovarus, the tibialis posterior muscle is transplanted to the anterior aspect of the foot, and the calcaneal tendon is elongated (Roaf and Hodkinson 1977). An advance stage of back-knee deformity, which causes the heel to lift off the ground, may require the achilles tendon of the affected leg to be lengthened.

Whenever the patient is walking, the nurse should attempt to support him from behind. Support should be especially directed to the prevention of hip hitching by the patient, and keeping the pelvis level. It will be easier to achieve this if the nurse is as tall as the patient. If the head and trunk are in correct postural alignment when his weight is shifted, the patient will walk, because it is an automatic response action (Parry and Eales 1976). In his early attempts at walking the patient might find it useful to gain support by using a broom, with a handle shortened to a suitable height. He can use it by holding it out in front of him, grasping the broom head in both hands. By keeping it in midline, it helps him maintain his balance. A rubber cap or ferrule should be fixed to the handle to give secure contact with the floor. Some patients may wish to use a walking stick, despite any postural disadvantages. When the patient's arm is hanging by his side, the correct height for the stick is with the top of the handle level with his wrist.

Walking and sitting will require the ability to turn. Turning can be accomplished by taking small steps towards the unaffected side. The patient should be instructed to turn by moving the affected leg forwards and the sound leg backwards (Parry and Eales 1976).

Stairs and stand-up exercises

If the patient can complete stand-up exercises, then climbing stairs should not present as much difficulty as may be thought. Negotiating stairs is only a problem for the patient who has been incorrectly taught. Also, the patient is often less afraid to climb stairs than to walk on the level, because the rise of the steps gives him the sensation of being less far from the ground (Hirschberg et al. 1976). Stepping-up exercises are usually practised in the physiotherapy department, but if no such facility is available, the nurse should take the patient to the bottom of a suitable flight of stairs, and explain what she wants him to do. Both patient and nurse may be surprised at what he can accomplish. Stair climbing has considerably greater exercise value than walking on the level, because it increases automatic co-ordination and control of the body.

The role of the occupational therapist

Occupation is a word which implies more than a person's actual employment. It includes the activity normally associated with the individual's environment, or his customary role in life. Occupational therapy often retains an 'arts and crafts' image. However, while such diversional activities have an important place in the management of the disabled, the occupational therapist is more concerned with assisting the patient to return to the fullest possible physical, mental and social competence of which he was previously capable. The activities which the therapist is concerned with include the following:

1   Mobility.

2   Personal care.

3   Domestic activities.

4   Work potential, including manual skills, work tolerance, and the ability to use educational skills.

5   Educational and recreational activities (Nichols 1976).

The occupational therapist is first concerned with an assessment of the patient's abilities, and then seeks methods and techniques to overcome his disabilities, sometimes by the introduction of aids and appliances.

She may also be able to conduct specific perceptual tests. One example may utilize a peg board, where the patient is asked to place pegs in a board that has a special arrangement of holes to eliminate guessing. If the patient continually fails to complete the test, he may be having difficulties with spatial differentiation. This may explain a patient who has difficulty in dressing, because he does not appreciate the relationship of different parts of clothing to his body, or cannot distinguish the right from the left side of the garment. Another test that can be done is to ask the patient to draw himself. The degree of distortion present might indicate the extent of alteration in his body image.

In the early stages of rehabilitation, the therapist will be likely to concentrate on activities designed to attempt to restore hand movement and to evaluate the patient's ability to carry out activities of daily living. However, return of full function to the arm is not usual. Even if gross movement returns, it is of little value to the patient, as the hand must be able to conduct finer action if it is to be useful again. Therefore, the patient may have to be retrained in one-hand activities, and will require adaptive devices to assist him (Policoff 1970, Moss 1981).

Peg boards and other exercises that demand the picking up and releasing of objects, will help to improve the fine coordination of the hand muscles. Large objects can be used initially and, as the patient improves, smaller objects such as draughts or dominoes can be substituted. These should be placed on an elevated board which demands maximum reach, and therefore elbow extension (Underwood 1974). Finally, the patient can be challenged to picking up and grasping pins (Rosenthal 1971).

Some patients are less likely to receive occupational therapy than physiotherapy and more likely to receive it later in the care process and to discontinue it earlier if progress is not made (Brocklehurst et al. 1978). Consequently, the nurse may have to provide for the patient, or assist him with, activities normally supported by an occupational therapist, e.g. dressing.

Dressing

The patient who does not need to wear a hospital gown or night attire should be dressed in his own day clothing. Being dressed in his own clothes not only seems to add to the patient's self-esteem, but also seems to reduce the incidence of incontinence (McCartney 1974). As well as a fair depth of spatial awareness, the activity of dressing calls for balance, coordination, reach, strength and dexterity (Nichols 1971).

Clothing should be selected with care. The nurse should advise the patient or relative to choose loose-fitting garments, with the minimum of fastenings, which will make them easier to put on and pull off. The fewer the number of garments required to preserve body heat the better. For example, an underskirt may not be necessary if a skirt is lined. A two-piece suit may be easier to put on than a dress and coat, while an anorak may be as warm as a man's jacket, but also more easily managed. Accessories, such as belts, braces and ties, should be kept to a minimum. Material should be chosen according to its ability to take the strains of transfer, and to be kept washed or dry cleaned if it becomes soiled, while still keeping its shape. Alterations might be usefully made to garments, e.g. by replacing small buttons with larger ones and enlarging button holes, or by replacing hook and eye fastenings with strips of Velcro.

The patient should be able to maintain a good sitting balance on the edge of the bed or in a chair before dressing activities begin. It might be helpful to begin the process with the patient learning how to undress. Undressing should begin by taking off the upper garment first, then the lower ones, and then shoes and socks. A button hook, elastic shoe straps and a long handled shoe horn may be helpful aids in this process. The patient should be taught to use the unaffected extremity first when undressing, and the affected limbs first when dressing. The dressing process should be planned, with items being laid out on the bed in the order in which they are to be put on.

The management of a few items of clothing might serve as useful illustrations.

Brassières usually cause a problem for female stroke patients. They can be altered so that they fasten with Velcro closures, and then slipped around the back of the patient. The affected arm should be placed through the shoulder straps first.

Vests, underslips and pullovers should be placed on the patient's lap, with the bottom of the garment towards his chest, and the front of the clothing facing downwards. The patient should then gather up the back of the garment, so as to be able to place the affected arm through the appropriate sleeve or opening. He should then pull the garment up the arm and over the shoulder. He is then asked to repeat the process on the unaffected side. Then, gathering the back of the garment, he should lower his head and pass the garment over it, pulling it down and adjusting as required.

For shirts, cardigans, coats and blouses, the affected arm is placed through the sleeve first, and then the garment is pulled over the shoulder, before being passed across the back of the neck. Then the unaffected arm is inserted, and the garment fastened. A dressing stick might help the patient to manipulate the garment across his back. This can be fashioned from a wooden single-bar coat hanger, from which the metal hook has been removed, with a rubber thimble attached to one end to cling to the material (Rudinger 1974).

The patient may prefer to put on his trousers while lying on the bed. Alternatively, he may prefer to put them on in a sitting position, just standing to pull them up around his waist. Zip fasteners should replace button flies.

Short stockings should have an elasticated opening which is easily stretched by one hand, so it can be pulled over the foot and stay in place, yet not impair the circulation of blood in the foot. Tights are extremely difficult for a female stroke patient to put on herself; nylons and a suspender belt which fastens like the brassière may be easier.

Intellectual impairment which interferes with dressing technique requires a systematic and critical approach from those caring for the patient, so that it may be overcome. Difficulties in remembering, loss of concentration and visual perceptive defects can be overcome in most cases, with patience and persistence. Any programme designed to help the patient relearn dressing technique may fail because of his inability to interpret what to move, or when, where and how to relate one object to another, e.g. an arm to the sleeve of a garment. Williams (1967) supports this assumption in her observations of the correlation deficiencies in visual motor copying ability and dressing activities. A relationship was observed between the ability to copy a series of three drawings, without gross error, and the patient's ability to perform dressing activity with the upper extremity. Patients unable to reproduce the drawings without errors seemed to have much difficulty in learning dressing habits.

Planning for dressing should involve both demonstration and verbal instruction. The identical procedure should be repeated each day, preferably with the same carer. Teaching a stroke patient to dress is a time-consuming procedure, so it is less likely to be successful if it is attempted on a busy hospital ward. It should either be delayed until staff can devote more time to the patient, or initiated in the occupational therapy department. Whenever possible, relatives should be involved, so that they can learn to avoid confusing the patient with an alternative technique. Relatives caring for the patient at home will have more responsibility in this area much earlier than if the patient is in hospital. The nurse must work out a technique which is realistic in relation to the abilities and intelligence of the family carers. More importantly, however, the dressing technique must be within the grasp of the patient, and he should be encouraged to dictate his preference in clothing, whenever possible. Dressing gives a great psychological boost to all patients; being able to dress oneself even more so. There is no excuse for a stroke victim being confined to wearing night attire for months, or even years. Even if a stroke patient is likely to spend the rest of his life in long-term care, if he can dress himself and is allowed to do so by nursing staff, the quality of his life can be improved. Nurses must begin to question their own attitudes towards dressing patients, which often include the false belief that it 'saves time', though in fact it is something contributing to the patient's dependency on them.

Shopping for clothing can be difficult for a stroke patient. A relative could identify the stores which sell a suitable range of products, and then a mutual arrangement may be possible with the management as regards access, and facilities for trying on clothing. This can lessen the stress of shopping for the patient. The use of a dressmaker or shopping from a catalogue are alternatives for the severely disabled, but the normal process of purchase helps to improve the social competence of the patient, which will help in raising his morale.

Travel and social contact

Few car drivers who suffer a major stroke are likely to be allowed to drive a motor car again. However, the majority of social functions demand travel in some form or another. Therefore, the social organization of the life of the patient demands the attention of nursing staff, if he is not to become isolated and withdrawn. The motivation of the patient to use private or public transport is the first factor to be considered. Using public transport and related facilities means coming into public view. The patient's willingness to expose his handicap depends on the degree of stigma which his stroke may hold for him.

Feelings of stigma, which may manifest themselves at the beginning of rehabilitation, impair the patient's motivation and, consequently, functional improvement during the programme. They also reduce the likelihood that he will be restored to his premorbid level of functioning, even months after the onset of stroke. Hyman (1971) claims that this poorer performance by stigmatized patients during rehabilitation appears to result from their aversion to one of the major goals, namely the resumption of social participation. Stigma possesses great explanatory power with respect to motivation and the patient's willingness to resume premorbid social roles. For a patient whose premorbid world was characterized by much social contact, a sense of stigma may make the regaining of such a world unappealing, and he will be reluctant to move outside the anonymity and security of home or hospital.

Stigma can be counteracted by the patient maintaining a positive self-concept, supported by family and staff. Over-protectiveness by the family may also act as a barrier to a functionally able patient moving back into society. However, the process of social isolation of stroke victims, and why it occurs, is by no means clear. A variety of explanations have been put forward. They include the possibility that the poor performance of patients who feel isolated is caused by the unattractiveness of the post-discharge way of life which awaits them (Hyman 1972). Another possible explanation is that isolated patients are deprived of the social support they require in the early stages of rehabilitation (Robertson and Swinn 1968).

There are physical as well as psycho-social impediments to travel and social contact, even for a patient who is fairly mobile. Public transport generally is in decline, and bus routes in particular are being cut back. This means that the stroke victim often has to walk considerable distances to and from bus stops. Some bus companies have introduced vehicles in which the driver can lower the step to within 4 inches of the ground, to accommodate disabled persons. Most trains, however, continue to demand that the passenger climb steep, narrow steps to gain access. Many public vehicles now have only one attendant, who both drives and collects fares and, therefore, is less likely to be in a position to offer assistance. No person likes to feel the psychological pressure of holding up busy commuter transport. The timing of journeys by public transport must be given attention, so that they can be geared to less busy periods. On country bus routes, the stroke victim might be helped by keeping to a regular timetable, so that transport personnel can become alert to his difficulties, and offer assistance.

Problems of travelling are not confined to vehicular access. Small physical movements present difficulties for stroke patients. Hodgins (1966), himself a stroke victim, described the effects of his catastrophe on his hand movements. He wrote, 'The loss of proprioceptive sense on the left side meant that the eye must watch and help control what the left hand was doing; it had no time to watch anything else. Loss of normal tactile sensation in the fingers of the left hand robbed the hand of its knowledge of accomplishment. Although the hand had good power and almost complete freedom of motion, the small muscles of the fingers were disobedient; thus [the hand] could not perform skilled acts.' Also, 'when the left hand stumbled, the right [unaffected] hand became confused'. Such physical impairment makes the handling of such small things as coins very difficult.

The assessment of the patient during the rehabilitation phase should include his ability to use public transport. There is a tendency for health care staff to leave such a development to the initiative of the patient and his family. The long-term goal of his mobilization programme must be complete integration within the community, and not confined to achieving mobility within the home.

References

Adams, G F (1971) Capacity after stroke, British Medical Journal, 1: 91

Amato, A, Hermsmeyer, C A and Kleinman, M (1973) Use of electromyographic feedback to increase inhibitory control of spastic muscles, Physical Therapy, 53 (10): 1063-1066

Anderson, T P (1970) Management of completed stroke, Oklahoma State Medical Association 63: 403-411

Bobath, B (1970) Adult Hemiplegia — Evaluation and Treatment, William Heinemann Medical

Brocklehurst, J C, Andrews, K, Richards, B, and Laycock, P J (1978) How much physical therapy for patients with stroke? British Medical Journal, 1: 1307-1310

Brudney, J et al. (1976) EMG feedback therapy — review of treatment of 114 patients, Archives of Physical Medicine and Rehabilitation, 57, Feb 55-61

Brunnstrom, S (1970) Movement Therapy in Hemiplegia, Harper & Row

Bucholz, C H (1911) On exercise treatment of paralysis, American Journal of Orthopedic Surgery, 9: 633

Casey, E B and Tupper, A D (1977) The neurologic patient, in S Mattingley (Editor), Rehabilitation Today, Update Books

Chuco, J (1971) Subluxation of the glenohumeral joint in hemiplegia, American Journal of Physical Medicine, 50: 139-143

Critchley, M (1931) Neurology of old age, Lancet, i: 1221-1230

Dardier, E L (1980) The Early Stroke Patient — Positioning and Movement, Ballière Tindall

Fay, T (1954) Basic considerations regarding neuromuscular and reflex therapy, Spastic Quarterly, 3, June: 5-8

Frenkel, H S (1890) Die therapie atactisher Bewegun störungen, Münchener Medicizinische Wochenschrift, 37:917

Fugl-Meyer, A R, Jääskö, L, Layman, I, Olsson, S and Steglind, S (1975) The post-stroke hemiplegic patient — a method of evaluation of physical performance, Scandinavian Journal of Rehabilitation Medicine, 7: 13-31

Garraway, W M, Akhtar, A, Prescott, R J and Hockey, L (1980) Management of acute stroke in the elderly — preliminary results of a controlled trial, British Medical Journal, 1: 1040-1043

Hewer, R L (1973) The management of hemiplegia, Proceedings of the Royal Society of Medicine 66, Sept: 882-884 (abridged)

Hirschberg, G G (1958) The use of stand up and step up exercises in rehabilitation, Clinical Orthopedics, 12:30

Hirschberg, G G, Lewis, L and Vaughan, P (1976) Rehabilitation, J B Lippincott

Hodgins, E (1966) Listen to the patient, New England Journal of Medicine, 274, (12): 657-661

Hollis, M (1976) Practical Exercise Therapy, Blackwell Scientific Publications

Hurwitz, L J and Adams, G F (1972) Rehabilitation of hemiplegia — indices of assessment and prognosis, British Medical Journal, 1: 94-98

Hyman, M D (1971) The stigma of stroke, Geriatrics, 26: 132-141

Hyman, M D (1972) Social psychological determinants of patient's performance in stroke rehabilitation, Archives of Physical Medicine and Rehabilitation, 53: 217-226

Jones, I (1974) Rehabilitation of a hemiplegic, Nursing Times, 70, Feb: 310-311

Kabat, H (1947) Studies on neuromuscular dysfunction XI — new principles of neuromuscular re-education, Permanante Foundation Medical Bulletin, 5: 3

Kabat, H and Knott, M M (1953) Proprioreceptive facilitation technics for treatment of paralysis, Physical Therapy Review, 33, Feb: 53-56

Kira, A (1967) The Bathroom, Bantam Books

Kratz, C (1978) Care of the Long-Term Sick in the Community, Churchill Livingstone

Kurasik, S and Sutton, B B (1969) Management of the hemiplegic stroke patient, Journal of the American Geriatrics Society, 17 July: 701-709

Licht, S (1970) Rehabilitation medicine, Archives of Physical Medicine and Rehabilitation, 51: 619

Licht, S (1975) A brief history of stroke and its rehabilitation, in S Licht (Editor), Stroke and Its Rehabilitation, Licht, E

McCartney, V C (1974) Rehabilitation and dignity for the stroke patient, Nursing Clinics of North America, 9: 693-701

McGilloway, F A (1980) The design process and nursing care, Nursing Mirror 151 (4): 34-5

McGinley, P (1959) Province of the Heart, Viking Press, p56

McNeil, F (1975) Stroke — nursing insights from a stroke-nurse victim, Registered Nurse, 38, Sept: 75-81

Mitchell, P (ed) (1977) Concepts Basic to Nursing, McGraw-Hill

Mitchell, P H, Ozuna, J and Lipe, H P (1981) Moving the patient in bed — effects on intracranial pressure, Nursing Research, 30, (4), July/Aug: 212-218

Moskowitz, E (1969) Complications in rehabilitation of hemiplegic patients, Medical Clinics of North America, 53, May: 54-59

Moskowitz, E, Lightbody, F E H and Freitag, N (1972) Long term follow up of the post stroke patient, Archives of Physical Medicine and Rehabilitation, 53: 167-172

Moss, B A (1981) What is occupational therapy? Nursing Times, 77, (41): 1769-1770

Nichols, P J R (1971) Rehabilitation of the Severely Disabled — Volume 2, Management, Butterworths

Nichols, P J R (1976) Rehabilitation Medicine, Butterworths

Oden, R (1918) Systematic therapeutic exercises in the management of paralysis in hemiplegia, Journal of the American Medical Association, 70: 828

Parry, A and Eales, C (1976) Handling the early stroke patient at home and in the ward, Nursing Times, 72: 1680-1683

Policoff, L D (1970) The philosophy of stroke rehabilitation, Geriatrics, 25, March: 99-107

Rantz, M J and Courtial, D (1978) Lifting, Moving and Transferring Patients, C V Mosby

Roaf, R and Hodkinson, L J (1977) The Paralysed Patient, Blackwell Scientific Publications

Rood, M (1954) Neurophysiological reactions as a basis for physical therapy, Physical Medicine Review, 34: 9

Rood, M (1962) The use of sensory receptors to activate, facilitate and inhibit motor response, automatic and somatic, in developmental sequence, in C Satterley (Editor), Approaches to the Treatment of Patients with Neuromuscular Dysfunction, W C Brown

Robertson, E K and Swinn, R M (1968) Determination of rate of progress of stroke patients through empathy measures of patients and family, Journal of Psychosomatic Research, 12, (3): 189-191

Rosenthal, A M (1971) Home management of the hemiplegic patient, American Family Physician, 3: 114-119

Rudinger, E (ed) (1974, revised 1976) Coping with Disablement, The Consumers Association

Schwartz, B (1968) The social psychology of privacy, American Journal of Sociology, 73: 741-752

Spencer, W A, Vallbona, C and Carter, R E (1965) Physiologic concepts of immobilization, Journal of Physical Medicine and Rehabilitation, 46: 90

Stern, P H, McDowell, F, Miller, J M and Robinson, M (1970) Efficiency of facilitation exercise techniques in stroke rehabilitation, Archives of Physical Medicine and Rehabilitation, 51: 526-531

Stryker, R P (1972) Rehabilitative Aspects of Chronic Nursing Care, W B Saunders

Tarling, C (1980) Hoists and Their Use, William Heinemann Medical

Todd, J M (1974) Physiotherapy in the early stages of hemiplegia, Physiotherapy, 60 (11): 336-342

Underwood, C S (1974) Occupational therapy in the early stages of hemiplegia, Physiotherapy, 60 (11): 342-345

van Itallie, P H (1970) Treatment trends — rehabilitating the stroke patient, Hospital Pharmacy, 5 (6): 26-32

Waddington, P J and Hollis, M (1980) Rules and mechanical principles, in Handling the Handicapped, Woodhead Faulkner, in association with the Chartered Society of Physiotherapists

Williams, N (1967) Correlation between copying ability and dressing activities in hemiplegia, American Journal of Physical Medicine, 46: 1332-1340

Williams, M and Lissner, H R (1969) Biomechanics of Human Motion, W B Saunders

CHAPTER 4

NURSING MANAGEMENT OF NUTRITION

Nutrition is a concept which implies scientific knowledge of the metabolic processes of cells, the constituents which form a quality diet and the relationships between nutrition, health, illness and disease. The nurse's assessment of the nutritional status of the patient will reflect the adequacy or otherwise of the patient's diet in supplying nutrients essential to life and well-being. Nutritional status will influence critically the therapeutic response of a patient to disease and disability. Many elderly people in particular tend towards a permanent state of subcritical malnutrition which lowers their ability to repair the effects of disease and injury in their body tissues (Exton-Smith et al. 1972).

Assessing food requirements

The need for food

Food is required for heat and energy. Heat is randomized energy in molecules of matter, and approximately 60% of all food energy obtained from diet is used to provide heat and thus maintain body temperature. Temperature is a measure of the extent of randomization in specific matter. The remaining 40% is used to provide energy, which can be defined as the power to do work. Only about 25% of all energy is used by the cells of the body (Wilson et al. 1979). The common heat unit in nutrition is the kilocalorie (kcal), which is the amount of heat required to raise the temperature of 1 kg of water by 1°C. The International Unit of heat is the joule (J).

$$1 \text{ kcal} = 4.184 \text{ kJ}$$

The need for energy

When man ingests, digests and absorbs food, the energy from the food is converted into adenosine triphosphate (ATP), which then serves as a source of energy for many energy-consuming cellular metabolic transformations (Figure 4.1). A side product of these activities is the generation of heat. The two main factors which determine the total energy need for an adult are basal metabolism and physical activity levels.

Figure 4.1 The need for energy

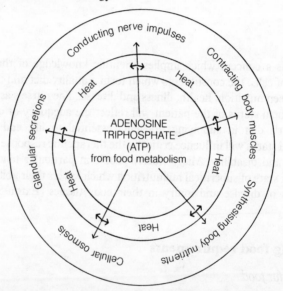

Basal metabolism is the minimum quantity of energy required, at all times, for the proper functioning of critical organs such as the brain, heart and liver, and for the maintenance of body temperature. Basal metabolism varies between individuals according to body size, body composition, age, sex, levels of endocrine secretion and health status, especially in cases involving fever and malnutrition. Although basal metabolism is usually measured from the ratio of height to weight, the nurse can make a rough calculation of energy requirements from weight alone, as follows:

Requirement per kilogram body weight per hour

	M	F
under 50 years of age	1.0	0.9 kcals/kg/hour
over 50 years of age	0.9	0.8 kcals/kg/hour

The equation for the basal metabolism for a patient under 50 years of age would be:

basal metabolism = 1 kcal (4.2kJ) or 0.9 kcal (3.8kJ) × body weight (kg) × 24 hours

while the equation for a patient over 50 years of age would be:

basal metabolism = 0.9 kcal (3.8kJ) or 0.8 kcal (3.4kJ) × body weight (kg) × 24 hours.

To convert body weight in pounds to body weight in kilograms, divide by 2.2.

Example   Using the above equation, the basal metabolic requirement for a 60 year old female who weighs 59kg (130lb), would be:

basal metabolism = 0.8 (kcal) × 59 (kg) × 24 (hours) = 1133 kcal (4740 kJ) for 24 hours

The type of tissue which composes the body will affect the basal metabolic requirement. Less energy is expended by fatty tissue than by muscle tissue. As women tend to have a higher percentage of fatty tissue in their body composition than men, their basal metabolic need is approximately 5% lower than that of men.

Basal metabolic requirements begin to decline in both sexes from the age of 20. By the time a man reaches the age of 75 his requirement is about 20% less than when he was a young man of 20.

When people are malnourished their basal metabolism is reduced. Several factors contribute to this, including a decrease in the amount of tissue requiring energy, a lower body temperature and decreased muscle tonicity. When the patient has a fever, the nurse should estimate that for every 0.5°C (1°F) above 37°C (98.6°F), the basal metabolism of the patient is increased by 7%. For example, when the temperature reaches 39.8°C (103.6°F), the metabolism of the body has increased by 35%.

The activity levels of the thyroid gland can have a dramatic effect on the basal metabolic requirements of the body. Amounts vary according to severity but hypothyroidism (myxoedema) can suppress the basal metabolism by 30-40%, while hyperthyroidism (thyrotoxicosis) can increase it by as much as 80%.

The energy needs of stroke patients, therefore, should be assessed in relation to body weight, body build, age, sex, health status and physical activity levels.

Physical activity   Different physical activities require different amounts of energy, e.g. three times more energy is required to walk up stairs than down. Early stroke victims may be classed as sedentary, but as activity levels increase so will energy requirements. Caloric expenditure not only depends on the type of activity being undertaken, but also on the intensity of the way in which it is being performed.

The recommended energy requirements for adults over 50 years of age, under normal circumstances are as follows:

Men: 2000 kcals/24 hours
Women: 1800 kcals/24 hours

The assessment

The assessment of the energy requirements of the stroke patient should be carried out by the nurse and/or dietician as soon as the life-threatening crisis has eased. The accuracy of such an assessment can never be exact, since there is no precise information on the minimum requirements of many nutrients and of various biochemical indices. Recommended dietary intakes tend to be defined to meet the needs of healthy persons, not individuals with health problems.

A periodic reassessment of energy requirements should be scheduled into the nursing care plan, according to the patient's progress. Too many calories and the patient will be likely to gain weight, which might inhibit mobility; too few and he will become undernourished and reluctant to exercise. If the patient suffers from obesity, a 1000 kcal reducing diet should be introduced immediately, with the agreement of the doctor and dietician. A good weight reduction diet should have the following characteristics:

1   It should satisfy all nutrient requirements except calories.

2   It should be kept as close as possible to the individual's tastes and habits.

3   The patient should maintain a sense of well-being, not feel fatigued and not suffer from hunger pangs between meals.

4   It should not be monotonous and uninteresting

5   It should be easy for the patient to obtain the constituents of the diet at home, or away from home.

The prevention, control and reduction of obesity in a stroke patient may be a larger problem for the nurse than preventing undernutrition or malnutrition. Malnutrition is not caused by simply taking too few calories, rather it is the result of a deficiency in the correct mixture of food constituents, vitamins and minerals.

Assessing the patient's appetite

Many stroke patients experience episodic loss of appetite. Failure to recognize and counteract these periods of anorexia can establish a vicious cycle of failure to eat, loss of energy and apathy towards food, with a lessening of the drive to eat, which will eventually lead to malnutrition. A decrease in the patient's appetite could result from one or more of the following factors:

Inability to control the chewing and swallowing of food

The muscles concerned with chewing and swallowing are likely to manifest the same degree of paralysis and loss of sensation as others throughout the affected side of the patient. Food which is pushed into the affected side of the mouth will cease to register as being there. Mastication becomes inefficient, and the patient requires more time to form a bolus from the food in his mouth. The tongue, itself a muscle, can lose the ability to pinpoint and recognize minute foreign bodies in the mouth, e.g. pips, grit and hair, and it becomes difficult for the patient to expel the unwanted entity without an accompanying amount of food. The patient can also experience difficulty controlling fluids, including the flow of saliva, without dribbling from the corner of his mouth on the affected side.

The physiology of swallowing involves a voluntary pushing of the food bolus upwards and backwards along the roof of the mouth, by the tongue. The soft palate lifts upwards, blocking off the opening to the nasal passages, so the food is directed through the nasopharynx towards the oesophagus. Paralysis of the soft palate could result in the unpleasant experience of nasal regurgitation, and an increased risk of choking.

As soon as possible, the patient should be encouraged to wear his dentures. If they are ill fitting, they should be replaced, and his mouth should be examined regularly for friction ulceration. Dental caries, if present, should receive early treatment, as tooth decay diminishes the ability to chew and enjoy food.

Loss of taste and smell

Ritchie (1960), relating his experience of being a stroke victim, explained how his senses of taste and smell were present or absent without any pattern becoming discernible, for a considerable period of time after his catastrophe. This affected his appetite and willingness to eat. Pleasant food smells stimulate the flow of secretions from the salivary glands, stomach lining and gall bladder, preparing the digestive organs for the reception of food. Salivary flow increases the ability of the taste buds on the tongue to function. Secretion flow results in stimuli registering at the cortical level as hunger.

A dirty, bad-tasting mouth decreases the appetite. Food can become trapped behind dentures, or in the affected side of the mouth. In addition, when a low fluid intake occurs, the first bodily reaction to conserve fluid is to decrease the saliva flow. Soft diets, which include a high percentage of milk or milk products, tend to coat the surface of the tongue, and subsequent bacilliary action can result in halitosis (foul-smelling breath).

Idiosyncratic preferences

In addition to the various physiological effects of taste and smell, common to all persons, each individual has his own food preferences. The appearance, taste, smell and texture of certain foods induce different effects among individuals. Causal factors include cultural and religious differences amongst peoples, and individual dietary experience. For example, the developments in food technology which may have come about since the life habits of the stroke patient were formed may not have stimulated any significant level of interest in him. The role of certain trace elements and vitamins in the diet may not be appreciated, or butter may be preferred to reinforced margarine because when the latter was invented it was seen as inferior to butter. New methods for food preservation, e.g. freeze drying, may be treated with suspicion, and there may be a tendency to prefer canned foodstuffs.

Emotional state

A stroke victim undergoes a wide range of emotional experience in relatively short periods of time. Shock, anger, denial, fear, frustration and depression alternate with hope, happiness, even occasionally euphoria. Such fluctuations in mood will have a direct effect on the patient's interest in food.

Visceral discomfort

Inadequate chewing and poor swallowing control can impose a greater burden on the mechanical activity of the stomach. Food which is ill cooked, or not too fresh, can induce gastritis, nausea and vomiting. This, if severe, can affect the fluid and electrolyte balance in the patient, as well as decreasing the appetite and subsequent food intake. Flatulence is frequently caused by the ingestion of large amounts of pulses, e.g. peas or beans, or by highly spiced foods. Constipation is also a cause of visceral discomfort, through an increase in peristaltic action in the colon.

The presence of pain (anywhere in the body)

Pain is a stimulus whereby the brain is alerted that an area of the body requires attention. It can be present as an acute, all-consuming stimulus which requires immediate intervention, e.g. angina, or as a subcritical prolonged discomfort, which interferes with everyday activities, e.g. arthritic pain. It is this persistent type of pain which is likely to induce a depressive reaction in the patient if uncontrolled, directing energy which can be ill afforded to sustaining the pain threshold. However, large amounts of analgesia can have a suppressive effect on the nervous system, which can reduce the desire to eat. Persistent pain increases the risk that large amounts of alcohol might be used in an attempt to obliterate cortical awareness of the pain. When taken in excess, alcohol acts as an appetite depressor, resulting in the development of vitamin deficiencies.

The presence of illness

The elderly are the group most at risk to stroke. They are usually the victims of multiple pathology as well. Therefore, the stroke patient can suffer a wide range of accompanying conditions, e.g. malabsorption syndrome, vitamin B_{12} deficiency anaemia etc, which may exacerbate the disability, or suppress the patient's ability to adapt to it. Illness of whatever type is usually associated with an increase in the body's demand for certain nutrients, e.g. protein for the repair of tissue. Protein deficiency seems to lead to a decreased inflammatory response to infection, and decreased ability of cells to resist bacterial and viral invasion, thereby increasing the risk of further illness.

A conscious effort to reduce eating

A wide range of factors which could contribute to a deliberate attempt by the stroke patient to reduce the amount or frequency of intake include economic factors, organic or other forms of mental illness, social isolation, guilt feelings related to dependency on others, and ignorance of the nutrients required and the foods which contain them.

Institutionalization

The factors mentioned above apply at the individual level of adjustment, in any situation. When the patient finds himself in a hospital or nursing home, he has to adapt to a more passive role, particularly as regards obtaining food. Any institution runs the risk of developing subcritical states of nutritional deficiency in patients. The quality of food purchased, the nutritional loss during storing, handling and cooking, and the imposition of restricted dietary choice can increase the risk of deficiency, particularly of iron and vitamins. Monotony in the diet adds to a depreciation in the attractiveness of food.

Whether or not one or more of these nine factors is assessed as contributing to a patient's loss of appetite, the nurse should remember that food habits, and feelings about food, are probably the major determinants of diet. Therefore, any assessment of the patient's nutritional requirements should include the following:

1 The quality of food normally eaten.
2 The quantity of food usually eaten.
3 The frequency of eating.
4 The rate of eating.
5 Adequacy of chewing and swallowing.
6 Food tolerance levels (Nordmark and Rohweder 1975).

The key words associated with such an assessment are that it should be systematic and conscious, not haphazard and intuitive. The eating habits and attitudes of a lifetime, despite the imposition of a stroke, will not be amenable to sweeping changes. Rather, there is a need to improve the quality of the patient's diet by making small deviations from food habits.

The patient's appetite can be increased in the following ways:

1 Getting the patient to think about food, especially foods that are enjoyed.
2 Heightening the patient's emotional state, e.g. his level of positive excitement.
3 Through the presence of pleasing food smells and food that looks attractive.

The nurse can achieve this by the following actions:

1   Providing a generally pleasant atmosphere and food attractively served.
2   Providing food at the preferred temperature, with seasoning according to taste, keeping in mind any medical restrictions such as low salt intake.
3   Eliminating any unpleasant sights, noises or smells.
4   Alleviating any physical discomforts, through correct positioning and careful timing of analgesia or other medications.
5   Providing for, and assisting the patient with, his oral hygiene.

Important nutrients in the stroke patient's diet

Carbohydrate and fibre

Approximately 45% of the total caloric intake of the patient is likely to be in the form of carbohydrate (Vir 1976). There have been suggestions that man's ability to metabolize carbohydrate is reduced with advancing age (Andres and Tobin 1972). Consequently, the search for alternatives results in up to one third of carbohydrate intake being of the refined type, i.e. sugar. Such a high percentage intake of refined carbohydrate results in a parallel reduction in fibre consumption. About 2g of dietary fibre is required daily by an adult, to give proper bowel habits by decreasing transit time and 'normalizing' stool consistency (Harvey et al. 1973). Fibre achieves these actions by increasing stool bulk and water-holding capacity which, in turn, reduces the risk of diverticular disease and colonic cancer by decreasing intraluminal pressure. Fibre consists of the structural components of plants, such as cellulose, hemi-cellulose and gums, which are for the most part indigestible by humans and have no food value in themselves. Examples of the fibre content of certain foodstuffs can be seen in Table 3.

Table 3 Examples of the fibre content of foodstuffs

Food	Total dietary fibre (g/100g)	Food	Total dietary fibre (g/100g)
Peas, frozen	7.8	Bread, brown	5.1
Beans, baked, canned	7.3	Bread, white	2.7
Carrots, boiled	3.7	Cereal, bran	44.0
Runner beans, boiled	3.4	Cereal, All-Bran	26.7
Brussel sprouts, boiled	2.9	Cereal, Puffed Wheat	15.4
Cabbage, boiled	2.8	Cereal, Shredded Wheat	12.3
Cauliflower, boiled	1.8	Cereal, Cornflakes	11.0
Lettuce, raw	1.5	Cereal, Special K	5.5
Tomato, raw	1.4	Cereal, Rice Krispies	4.5
Bread, wholemeal	8.5		

When a very soft diet is offered to a stroke patient, a teaspoonful of bran should be sprinkled over the most appropriate foodstuff once or twice a day. Many proprietory brands of dietary additives are available, but they tend to put the patient to unnecessary expense, while bran is easily available.

Amino-acids and protein

Evidence regarding the exact need for protein and individual amino-acids is conflicting. Suggested requirements range from 0.35—0.9 g/kg body weight, per 24 hours. Eight amino-acids must be present in the diet for the body to synthesize protein. The eight are phenylalanine, tryptophan, methionine, lycine, leucine, isoleucine, valine and threonine. Animal proteins contain all eight essential amino-acids. Vegetable proteins are deficient in some, but if a mixture is taken, one may supplement the other. For example, a mixture of maize and beans can provide a strict vegetarian with adequate protein.

Protein-rich foods help to alleviate a negative nitrogen imbalance, which can occur in the stroke patient through an increase in urinary nitrogen excretion caused by immobility. This depletes the stores of nitrogen required for protein synthesis, which is essential for tissue repair. The average adult has a turnover of approximately 300 g/day. The energy cost of daily protein synthesis is put at 2000 kJ, or about 30% of the basal metabolic expenditure (DHSS 1976). Such calculations neglect, however, any energy involvement in the breakdown of proteins in health or illness.

Fats

Because the body can synthesize fat from carbohydrate and protein, dietary fat is not essential to life. Fats are composed of fatty acids and glycerol, and are classified according to the amount of saturated or unsaturated fatty acid present. Saturated fats, e.g. butter, when taken in excessive amounts are said to play a part in the development of atherosclerosis. Consequently, the stroke patient should be encouraged to change to unsaturated fat, e.g. margarine, instead of butter, and corn oil for cooking. Dietary fat, in large amounts, should be discouraged, because of its high caloric component. For example, 30 g (1 oz) of butter gives 226 kcals, compared with 112 kcals for the same amount of sugar.

Low fat foods include the following:

chicken	liver
plaice	cottage cheese

cod

tea and coffee

Bovril

jam and honey

bread and cereals

fruit and vegetables

sugar and boiled sweets

marmalade

Foods which should be discouraged because of their high fat content include the following:

herring

mackerel

salmon

nuts

biscuits

cream crackers

pastries

cream

cream cheese

pork

duck

goose

chocolate

ice cream

Vitamins

In normal health, an adequate diet will supply all the vitamins which the body requires, and there is no need for supplementation. However, a study carried out by Exton-Smith et al. (1972) showed that housebound elderly persons tended to be deficient in vitamins C and D. Foods high in water-soluble vitamin C tend to be those which, in the raw state, the stroke patient finds difficult to chew, and which when cooked lose much of their vitamin C content. An alternative method of providing vitamin C in the diet of a stroke patient is the giving of unsweetened natural fruit juice as part of the daily diet. The adult requirement of vitamin C is 20 mg daily. See Table 4 for examples of the vitamin C content of some foodstuffs.

Table 4 Examples of vitamin C content in foodstuffs

Food	Vitamin C (mg/100g)
Orange	50
Grapefruit	40
Apple	5
Grape, white	4
Tomatoes, raw	20
Brussel sprouts, boiled	35
Cabbage, boiled	20

A low dietary intake of vitamin D, in conjunction with a lack of synthesis of the vitamin through exposure to sunlight, can present additional problems for the stroke patient. Inadequate levels of vitamin D increase the risk of the development of osteomalacia i.e. skeletal rarefaction, or loss of density in bone. Osteomalacia increases the risk of fracture when a fall occurs, thereby compounding the mobility problems of the patient.

While vitamin D is not destroyed by normal cooking methods, it is not widely distributed in foodstuffs. Fish-liver oils, in liquid or capsule form, are perhaps the best source of this vitamin. When the stroke patient is housebound, vitamin D supplements should be given by this method, or by fortified margarine. The recommended adult intake of vitamin D is 400 International Units daily.

While the nervous system requires all the various vitamins for its development, subsequent maintenance of its integrity and function rests with the vitamin B group, and in particular vitamin B_1, which is also known as thiamine. Subclinical thiamine deficiency could result in symptoms such as loss of appetite, general lethargy, insomnia and increased irritability in the patient. More serious deprivation can lead to destruction of parts of the central and peripheral nervous systems, causing serious and frequently irreversible dysfunction (Dreyfus 1979). Consequently, thiamine deficiency in the stroke patient should be avoided. For every 1000 kcal in the diet it is recommended that 0.4 mg of thiamine be present. Examples of thiamine content of certain foodstuffs can be seen in Table 5.

Table 5 Examples of foods with a high thiamine content

Food	Thiamine (mg/100g)
Ham, boiled	0.50
Liver, fried	0.30
Peas, boiled	0.25
Bread, wholemeal	0.20
Bread, with vit. B_1 added	0.18
Milk	0.04

Iron

Iron-deficiency anaemia is the most likely cause of anaemia in the stroke patient, either in hospital or at home. The commonest cause is a low dietary intake of iron, but compounding this is the degree to which the patient may have developed achlorhydria, i.e. a decrease in gastric secretion, which is a normal manifestation of advancing age. The patient with achlorhydria is less able to absorb the iron which is present in the diet. In a healthy male weighing 70 kg, the total body iron is approximately 4.2 g. 60% of this is present in the haemoglobin of the red blood cell, or erythrocyte. In women almost all the body iron is present in the red blood cells. The bulk of remaining iron, approximately 800 mg in men and 250 mg in women, is present in muscle myoglobin. This represents the oxygen-storing capacity of muscle, which allows it to contract, and lack of which results in muscle fatigue (Heinrich 1975). Iron is also stored in the liver and bone marrow.

About 1 mg of iron is lost daily from the gastro-intestinal tract. Iron from foods of animal origin tends to be absorbed better than that from foods of plant origin, including iron from various cereals and breads (Larisse 1975). Iron from vegetable origin is better absorbed when eaten with meat or fish. Consequently, stroke victims whose ethnic origins demand a vegetarian diet, e.g. Moslems, for whom rice and chapattis sometimes constitute the bulk of the diet, are more at risk to iron-deficiency anaemia than others. However, the recycling of iron by the body, and the subsequent small daily loss, means that simple iron-deficiency anaemia is not likely to occur in the absence of other pathology or dietary mismanagement.

Calcium

Immobilization caused by paralysis and enforced bedrest invariably results in the occurrence of osteoporosis, which is a disturbance in the total volume of skeletal bone, with change in its composition. It causes atrophy of both the protein matrix and osseous content of bone, resulting in calcium imbalance. The integrity of bone is normally maintained by a combination of weight bearing and tension on the origins and insertions of muscles, which result from motion and activity. Weight bearing and calcium dietary supplements are not enough to prevent osteoporosis developing. Changing the gravitational position of the stroke patient does not significantly diminish calcium loss either. Only restoration of muscle strength, or the presence of muscle pull due to spasticity in the stroke patient, can arrest osteoporotic changes caused by disuse (Hirschberg et al. 1976). In the course of time, as activity increases, the osteoporotic changes will slow down and calcium loss will diminish. The nurse can help the patient as follows:

1   Encouraging him to adopt an upright position for part of the day.

2   Instituting passive and active range-of-motion exercises two or three times a day.
3   Mobilizing the patient as quickly as possible.

Fluids

The approximate normal fluid balance for an adult in 24 hours can be stated:

Intake	*Output*	
2000 ml from food and fluids	2000 ml:	1000 ml from 'invisible loss (i.e. respiration, perspiration, faeces) 1000 ml from urinary output

Urinary output varies with fluid intake and perspiration levels. To achieve a correct balance, the stroke patient on a normal diet should drink a minimum of eight cups of fluid a day. The remaining need will be met from the fluid constituent of food. An adequate fluid intake is essential to maintain good oral hygiene and to prevent urinary tract infections, excessive loss of calcium in the urine and an increase in the viscosity of the blood, which in turn increases the risk of thrombus formation.

Idiosyncratic preferences play an important role in the amount and type of beverage consumed. There is a wide variety of preference associated with even the common beverages such as tea and coffee. For example, some prefer their tea or coffee hot or iced, according to season, while milk, cream, lemon, sugar and saccharin vary in presence and amount. Preferences are not easily maintained on admission to hospital. Inadequate intake in hospitalized stroke patients could result from low staffing levels, or routinized deployment of available staff. In an attempt to cope with such problems, nurses may standardize the choice of beverage offered the patient. However, the nurse who presents an elderly stroke patient with a glass of orange squash on a winter's morning should not be too surprised if only an occasional sip is taken.

If a nurse does not have time to prepare a preferred beverage, or policy prohibits the relative preparing it in the ward kitchen, the relative might be encouraged to bring it to the hospital in a vacuum flask or other container from the hospital cafeteria or concession area, after seeking the nurse's advice regarding any medical restriction. As soon as the patient's condition allows, relatives should be encouraged to take the patient to the concession area for a beverage.

There is no reason why alcohol should not be tolerated in small amounts, providing there is no possibility of any adverse reaction involving the patient's chemotherapy regime. A glass of sherry, wine or stout before, or with, a meal, can help the patient's appetite, and increase the overall calorie intake. A drink before bedtime may help promote relaxation and sleep. Low-calorie and non-alcoholic lagers are now available as alternatives.

Problems associated with obtaining, cooking and presenting food

Obtaining food

In the early stage of rehabilitation the stroke patient must rely almost totally on others. Relatives, neighbours, home helps and voluntary service workers are the main suppliers of food for housebound patients. Hospitals are faced with a moral responsibility to provide adequate nutrition for the patient, even at times of disruption resulting from industrial disputes. The problem of the housebound patient is more complex. The modern social trend of depopulating city centres, and providing housing in estates on the periphery of towns, is slowly being reversed as transport costs rise. The problems of the housebound are compounded as the number of small, corner shops, which stocked a large variety of food and other household materials, decrease and are replaced by hypermarket complexes. Consequently, the stroke patient who is unable to drive a car, secure a lift from others or use a diminishing public transport system, will have difficulty in obtaining a reliable supply of groceries and other materials. The cost of hiring a taxi is now beyond the budget of most disabled persons.

While the stroke patient has to rely on others to do his shopping, it is important that the nurse takes time to discuss with the shopper the kind of foodstuffs which should be purchased, within the restrictions of the patient's budget and preference. The patient may be reluctant to offer such advice in case the shopper withdraws his help. The following basic foods should be included in the patient's diet each day:

At least 300 ml ($\frac{1}{2}$ pint) milk
One helping meat or fish.
One egg.
Four slices of bread, wholemeal if possible.
30 g (1 oz) margarine.

One helping potatoes.
One helping other vegetables or fruit.
Eight cups preferred beverage.

Against adverse situations, the patient should be encouraged to keep an emergency food store. This might include tins of baked beans, fruit, vegetables, soups, evaporated milk, corned beef, sardines and so on. The nurse should check that this emergency stock is replaced periodically in order to prevent spoilage through ageing.

Meals-on-wheels is a well publicized local authority service which provides a balanced meal, usually two or three times a week, for elderly, housebound persons. However, people who are eligible often do not use this service because:

1   It is seen as a charity.
2   Organizational restraints may mean that delivery time may not suit the individual.
3   Dietary preference and physiological deficits are not easily catered for.

As an increase in mobility occcurs, and the patient begins to regain his independence, the shopping habits acquired over a lifetime will tend to govern the way he buys food, and the type he buys. Daily shopping at the local shop is still the practice of most elderly citizens. Many still have no refrigerator, which restricts the choice of food, e.g. canned foods instead of fresher frozen ones. A telephone can be useful to place an order at a local store, or a relative or neighbour might be willing to leave a grocery list at the shop for delivery. A small extra charge is usually involved, but an increasing number of stores are ceasing to operate such a service altogether. In rural areas a grocery van service is still to be seen bringing the 'shop' to the isolated household, but again, increasing fuel costs are resulting in the disappearance of such services.

Modern methods of packaging fresh foods may present problems for the stroke patient. Bacon, other meats and cheese, for example, should be bought from the block rather than prepackaged. An electric can opener can be helpful to a stroke patient who relies heavily on canned foods. When bottles or jars have screw tops, and contents are likely to be consumed quickly, it can be helpful if the tops are loosened slightly before shelving, so the patient can cope with opening them. Milk should be purchased in bottles rather than cartons, which sometimes test the manipulative skills of the ablest person.

In procuring food for a stroke patient, whether in hospital or home, it is important to remember that to persons accustomed to a traditional diet, be it a Western diet or otherwise, certain constituents of the diet may have a psychological importance out of proportion to their nutritional value.

Cooking and presenting food

The importance of taste and smell for the maintenance of the patient's appetite has been discussed earlier. Equally important is the appearance of food as an energy-intake regulator. Most people associate high volume diets with high caloric intake. Stroke victims may have to adjust the volume/frequency ratio of their intake for a while, if not permanently. When the volume of the diet decreases the patient should be reassured that his nutritional needs are being met. He will be encouraged if he is offered food which is properly cooked, is served at the right temperature and looks good to eat. Diets consisting mostly of liquids can be extremely boring, and the patient will lose interest very quickly. Small frequent meals are peferable to large ones, and a heavy evening meal should be avoided, to reduce the risk of obesity developing.

The cooking of food in hospital is outside the control of the nurse and the patient. While the patient is in hospital, however, the occupational therapist has an important role in teaching him how to prepare simple meals in spite of his disability. Several types of aid can be provided to enable the patient to cope with such everyday tasks as buttering bread. For cooking in the home, electricity presents fewer problems than does gas. If the patient has a gas cooker, a battery operated lighter should be used, rather than matches, to light it. Heavy-based pans can reduce the movement of the pan on the cooker as the hemiplegic patient stirs or turns the food. If the patient becomes easily tired while standing, a wide-based high stool might provide support.

Basic principles of hygiene should not be neglected in food preparation just because the patient has a disability. The nurse should take any opportunity to observe the patient's ability to cope with hygiene, and offer realistic advice when appropriate. Waste-disposal methods used by the patient should also be checked to see if they represent a health risk.

The method by which food is presented to the patient is of critical importance to whether or not it will be eaten. It can either support or undermine the adult integrity of the patient, diminish or improve and bolster his self-image. Habits associated with dining have become increasingly informal in recent years with the introduction of snack meals, take-aways etc. For the stroke patient, it is necessary that crockery is used whenever possible, and that it is placed on a firm base, be it a table, bedtable or tray, and not balanced precariously on his knees. Ideally the base should be just above waist high, and about 4 inches away from the patient's chest, in order to keep the distance from the plate to the mouth within his control. When sitting out of bed the patient's chair should offer adequate support to the back and lower part of the body, to enable him to achieve the rocking movement associated with eating. Insecurity pushes the patient into attempting to bring the food the full distance from the plate, rather than following the normal eating action of meeting it partway.

The hospital nurse should obtain non-slip mats and plate guards from the occupational therapy department for transfixing the crockery (Figure 4.2).

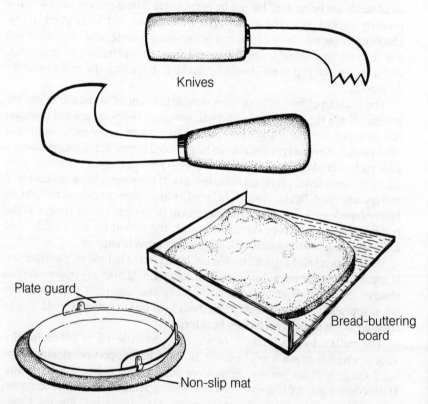

Knives

Plate guard

Bread-buttering board

Non-slip mat

Figure 4.2 Feeding aids

Specially designed, all-in-one utensils are also available, and should be used in preference to spoons, as soon as the patient can cope. The main part of the meal should never be offered in a high-sided soup or desert dish. Plastic tumblers should be used instead of drinking glasses in the early stages of rehabilitation, while straws that bend are useful for giving those patients who can cope with them a greater sense of control over liquids. Spouted, plastic beakers also help the patient control the flow of liquids in his mouth, but it is important for the resocialization of the patient that he begins to gain confidence in manipulating a cup as soon as possible.

In the early stages of recovery, food is almost bound to go astray between plate and mouth. Spillages can inhibit the patient's willingness to persevere with feeding himself. A washable, plastic placemat should be placed on the table or tray and, if he is ambulant, he should be placed at a table, where the floor can easily be cleaned if spillage should occur. The nurse ought to ensure that all those likely to attend the patient, whether in hospital or home, refrain from commenting on any spillage, and present an attitude of acceptance. Sarcastic or degrading remarks will only increase the patient's sense of worthlessness and feelings of being a burden to others. Positive comments about the patient's progress should be encouraged.

Paper tissues are a cheap and disposable alternative to table napkins. A number of loose tissues should be placed on the table at the unaffected side of the patient, and a paper bag attached to the arm of the chair, or table, on the same side as a receptacle.

A case conference between nursing staff, dietician and occupational therapist can help to solve the individual problem of the patient.

The food presented to the patient should contain all the nutrients suggested as being essential, but efforts will be wasted if food is offered in a way that increases the likelihood of its rejection. The appropriate temperature of food is difficult to maintain in a hospital environment, but it can be aggravated if the nurse offers the patient more food than he can cope with in a reasonable period of time. Slowness in chewing and swallowing means that the food on his plate will get cold quickly. A small portion of each type of hot food should be offered initially, while the remainder is kept warm in the kitchen of the ward, or home. Courses should be kept separate until the patient has finished each one. Food on the plate should be kept separate by careful placement. If soup dishes are used for the main course, the food will tend to merge together, presenting an unappetizing mess, especially if gravy is then added. Even food which has to be cut up for the patient can be arranged so as to have an attractive appearance. Most people enjoy a glass of water, milk or wine with their meal, with any hot beverage kept to the end.

Time is one of the most important dietary factors with the stroke patient. Time to consider what he wants to eat, how and in what order he wants it, and time to eat it. The disorganization of his cognitive processes can make decision-taking difficult, and the verbalized result may be reversed. Because of this, the nurse or family should be aware that the answers to questions can come out wrong. For example, if the question is, 'Do you want a second helping Mr Jones?', the patient may wish to say 'Yes, please', but the answer comes out as 'No', and the second helping disappears, to the frustration of the patient. In the hospital ward, time presents a greater pressure on the patient than at home. Other patients finish their food in normal time, dishes are being cleared away, to fit in with the domestic worker's schedule, and unconscious pressure is placed on the patient to conform to the speed of others. If the nurse feels the patient is being pressurized into saying he is satisfied, she should leave foods such as bread and butter, fruit or biscuits at hand, and discuss the problem with those concerned.

Feeding the patient

Stroke patients will frequently need to be fed by the nurse or relative, especially in the early stages following their catastrophe. Such a period of dependence should be kept to a minimum. Sommerville (1968) wrote:

> It is incredible how many patients are allowed to leave hospital completely dependent from an ADL point of view. For months the junior nurse has cut up their food and even fed them when cooperation between nursing staff and occupational therapists would have resolved their problem in a matter of weeks or even days.

Feeding a patient, while encouraging his independence, requires the skill of an experienced nurse, and the task should not be left to inexperienced and unskilled workers.

In preparation, the nurse should ensure the patient's mouth is clean, and if he uses dentures, that they are securely in place. Whenever possible she should adopt a supervisory role, encouraging the patient to help himself, yet ready to intervene as soon as he indicates he is tired, or is becoming frustrated with his efforts. Before starting to feed the patient the nurse should ensure she has all the requirements to hand. She should remain seated throughout, in a position which keeps unnecessary movement to a minimum. It is useful to use paper tissues as napkins to protect the patient's clothing. Plastic bibs, however helpful from the nurse's point of view, are degrading to the patient, and should never be used. Whenever possible the patient should direct the order and amounts in which the food is offered. The nurse should start by offering small amounts to the unaffected side of the patient's mouth. She should encourage him to wipe away any dribbling, and check periodically that food is not trapped in the affected side of the mouth before increasing the size of the portions. The patient should be directed to explore the affected side of his mouth with his tongue to dislodge trapped food. Eating is an important socializing opportunity for the patient, and even the aphasic patient should be encouraged to demonstrate responsiveness, verbal or otherwise. When the meal is finished, the patient may need to rest for a short while before the nurse attends to his oral hygiene by offering a mouthwash, or helping him to clean his dentures. Stroke patients have a very low fatigue threshold, and the nurse must not rush the pace of care.

A food diary is a very useful tool for the patient, or his family. It offers a written record of progress, and where such progress is normally slow, it can be reinforcing to all concerned to realize what actual progress has been made. It also gives day-to-day stimulus to learning the constituents of adequate nutrition, and encourages creativity and innovation in the feeding process. It also offers the professional the opportunity to offer appropriate and realistic advice, and if the diary is filled in honestly, feedback that the advice has been understood. The headings used in the diary would be for the individuals involved to choose. Examples could include date, time, type of food or drink consumed, amount of food taken or left, and any difficulties involved in cooking, presenting or consuming food.

Medications

Stroke patients often have to take medication for reasons of prevention as well as cure. Hemiplegia renders it extremely difficult for the patient to unscrew the bottle top and select a single pill, or pull a cork, and pour liquid with control. In addition, visual disturbances may render reading the label difficult. In the home, it is useful to buy a number of cheap, coloured egg cups, and write in large letters on each one the time medication is to be taken. If the patient has difficulty reading the time, he can differentiate by the colour of the egg cup. If the patient has to be left alone for a time, the correct medication can be left in the egg cup, decreasing the risk of him consuming multiple doses, and enabling the relative to see if he has taken it or not. Bottles of medicine should not be left at the bedside at night. Because medicines come in many shapes and sizes, advice may be needed as to the easiest way to take them, for example whether liquid alternatives are available, or if capsule contents can be scattered on food.

Food and socialization

The process of consuming food is a well-conducted social institution. The social stimulation of taking food is a key part of the sensory perceptual environment of all individuals. Food is important to our social as well as our physical well-being. For Western populations food is no longer dominated by the primitive urge of survival. Rather, this urge has become merged with the realization of social needs and eating has become dominated by the clock, e.g. 'the lunch hour'. The presentation of food and drink to business colleagues is considered to be a necessary part of mercantile life. Housewives can be seen chatting over coffee after shopping, in a café or in the home. It is considered impolite in most cultures not to offer a visitor a cup of coffee, or other refreshment. Therefore, the ability to offer or receive such symbolic offerings affects our social position within the different groups in our society. The stroke patient has to overcome his disability in order to be able to re-enter this system again, otherwise he risks social isolation. He must overcome his embarrassment, and avoid inducing embarrassment in others. At first the patient is likely to want to avoid all visitors and refuse all invitations. The family members will play the vital role in helping him overcome this reticence. As soon as he feels confident in coping with a cup or glass, relatives or neighbours, who can be relied on to be positive in their approach to any mishaps, should be invited for coffee or tea. When the patient can cope with and enjoy this situation, and providing he is making parallel progress in other areas, he should be encouraged to accept an invitation outside the home. When the patient is invited to a dinner group, certain arrangements could be made with the hosts beforehand, e.g. what type and amount of food the patient can cope with, the placement of cutlery, provision of napkins etc. A secret signal could be arranged with the patient to inform him if he is dribbling food from the corner of the mouth. Toilet arrangements constitute an important part of all social gatherings. The invitation may be refused simply because the patient is afraid he will not be able to get to a lavatory in a particular home or building. Whenever possible, discreet arrangements might be made with the hosts for the patient to have the opportunity to use a receptacle brought by the relative, and for the disposal of the contents, with minimum disruption to the proceedings.

Many relatives and patients would find it difficult and embarrassing to discuss such matters, even within the family circle. The nurse can play a useful role as group leader, or intermediary, in any discussions associated with such difficulties, enabling those who will give or receive hospitality to have a chance to explore the problem, and find their own solutions.

If the patient is to retain or return to some form of employment, his ability to cope with the social aspects of eating will dictate the type of work he can do, and the level of acceptance or rejection by those he would be working with. Failure to cope could lead to feelings of uselessness and stigma, isolating the patient perhaps to the extent of him becoming what Goffman (1971) described as a 'non-person', someone who is ignored in any social interaction in that they take neither the role of the performer, nor of audience. Food and the social importance of eating form helpful tools which the nurse can use to prevent such a situation developing.

References

Andres, R and Tobin, J (1972) Proceedings of the 9th International Congress of Gerontology, 1: 276

DHSS (1976) Research and Obesity — A Report of the DHSS/MRC group, HMSO

Dreyfus, P M (1979) Nutritional disorders of the nervous system, in R Hodges (Editor) Nutrition — Metabolic and Clinical Applications, Plenum Press, pp. 53-81

Exton-Smith, A N, Stanton, B R and Windsor, A C M (1972) Nutrition of Housebound Old People, King Edward's Hospital Fund for London

Goffman, E (1971) The Presentation of Self in Everyday Life, Penguin

Harvey, R F, Pomare, E W and Heatson, K W (1973) The effects of increased dietary fibre on intestinal transit, Lancet, i: 1278

Heinrich, H C (1975) Definition and pathogenesis of iron deficiency, in H Kief (Editor) Iron Metabolism and its Disorders, American Elsevier, pp. 113-122

Hirschberg, G G, Lewis, L and Vaughan, P (1976) Rehabilitation — A Manual for the Care of the Disabled and Elderly, J B Lippincott

Larisse, M (1975) Dietary iron absorption, in H Kief (Editor), Iron Metabolism and its Disorders, American Elsevier, pp. 25-33

Nordmark, M T and Rohweder, A W (1975) Scientific Foundations of Nursing, 3rd edition, J B Lippincott

Ritchie, D (1960) Stroke — A Diary of Recovery, Faber & Faber

Sommerville, J G (1968) Rehabilitation of the hemiplegic patient, Rehabilitation, 164: Jan-Mar: 5-9

Vir, S C (1976) Dietary intake and nutritional status of institutionalised and non-institutionalised aged, PhD thesis, Queen's University, Belfast

Wilson, E D, Fisher, K H and Garcia, P A (1979) Principles of Nutrition, 4th edition, J Wiley & Sons

CHAPTER 5

NURSING MANAGEMENT OF ELIMINATION

Introduction

While much of what is included in this chapter apertains to other groups of patients, it is of such critical importance to the stroke patient that detail cannot be regarded as abstruse.

Little and Carnevali (1976) claim that many of the statements of assessment which nurses make project the nurse's problems in coping with the patient and turn them into the patient's problems. They also claim that the patients most at risk in this instance include those:

1 Who take up more time than nurses feel they have available.

2 Whose way of communicating with nursing staff is not acceptable.

3 Who are dull and uninteresting, but due to stay around for a long time.

4 Who are in an emotional state that is communicable, and causes discomfort, uneasiness or outright hostility in others.

On such criteria a stroke patient, particularly one who is aphasic and incontinent, must be seen as being at high risk to be viewed as a 'nursing' or 'incontinent' problem.

The word 'incontinent' has serious negative connotations for patients and relatives, as well as health care staff. Such connotations will, in turn, indirectly affect the approach of the staff, and the motivation of the patient, toward his regaining social reliability. What might be a temporary loss of skill may be changed into a permanent aberration, simply by poor management resulting from negative attitudes.

Chamber's dictionary offers two definitions of the word 'incontinence'. First, 'not restraining the passion or appetites', and second, 'unable to restrain the natural discharges or evacuations of the body'. While the second definition is now universally accepted, it is worth remembering that the former, older definition may cause additional distress when applied to an elderly patient. They may see it as an implicit comment on their morality. Indeed, the word 'incontinence' should be used with extreme care, or avoided altogether, in conversation with patients and relatives.

Most nurses will be aware of, and concerned about, the problems of urinary and faecal incontinence in their patients. After all, coping with the results of incontinence consumes many working hours, and is extremely costly in laundry services and equipment, as well as being generally unpleasant for all concerned. Most importantly, it may be the deciding factor in whether the patient goes home or is placed in long-term care. In spite of this situation, there remains a paucity of nursing literature and research in the subject. Even booklets which are specially prepared to inform and support the stroke victim and his family give comparatively little space to this problem (e.g. Mulley 1978). On the whole, medical practitioners tend not to be interested in the subject, except in relation to special procedures associated with surgery. Isaacs (1979) claims that, by failing to cope with incontinence, the health service is failing its most needy patients. While it is generally accepted that the inability to control the flow of urine is one of the most devastating social disasters that can affect anyone, the problem of incontinence, especially amongst the elderly and long-term sick, has been left to the jurisdiction of the nurse.

However, nurse education practices, particularly at the preregistration level, do not appear to have responded to this challenge. The few education hours associated with the subject tend to centre on 'coping' with the problem, and on preventing the occurrence of additional complications, such as pressure sores. This is particularly unfortunate in view of the fact that in hospitals it is usually the junior learners who have to 'cope' with the results of incontinence. Theoretical instruction and skill developed through bowel or bladder retraining programmes invariably centre in a few specialized wards, or with a few interested individuals. Retraining skills among nurses are not generally apparent in all wards of a hospital where such patients might be found, including acute medical wards. In the community, until mandatory training was introduced for district nurses in Britain, the development of retraining skills was variable and haphazard, because the framework just was not there. Consequently, while it could have been expected that the nursing profession would have assumed a proficiency in the care of the incontinent patient, this is not apparent. According to Willington (1975), 'the need to provide a solution to the problem is often sacrificed so the needs of the ward as a whole can be maintained'. From observing the care offered stroke patients, Patrick (1973) claims that nurses did not help the patient meet basic elimination needs, or appear to understand the special needs of these patients. Special training has been found to be necessary to alert nurses to such needs, and to improve the attitude of nursing staff towards stroke patients (Hamerin 1982).

The numbers of stroke patients who will be likely to suffer incontinence cannot be ascertained. It will depend on the severity of their stroke, the location of the lesion, the presence of other relevant pathology and any emotional trauma which the patient may have suffered. Age alone does not appear to be a factor (Willington 1969), although the normal biological degeneration associated with ageing will compound the problem. For example, there would be more likelihood of reflex voiding, or loss of bladder tone, leading to more frequent and smaller urinary evacuations, with a consequent shortening of the waiting period.

There is no apparent difference between the sexes as to the likelihood of incontinence after stroke (Isaacs and Walkey 1964, Brocklehurst et al. 1968). The stroke patient is more likely to develop urinary than faecal incontinence. The latter is more likely to be the result of poor nursing management, or the confused mental state of the patient, rather than cortical disruption of nerve impluses.

Nursing assessment

An accurate history of the patient's previous habits of elimination will form the cornerstone of his care. Such a history should include the following information:

1 The usual time of day for bowel movement.

2 The frequency of micturition, including any desire to pass urine at night (nocturia). (If a stroke patient must use the toilet at night, this may have implications for his safety, especially in the home.)

3 Any difficulties with either bowel movements or micturition, e.g. the presence of haemorrhoids or an enlarged prostate gland in a male patient may create pain, loss of blood or difficulty initiating urinary flow.

4 The usual dietary constituents, including an estimation of the roughage or

fibre in the diet, and the usual mealtimes of the patient.

5   The usual level of fluid intake, and its distribution over a 24 hour period.

6   Usage of laxatives.

In addition, an enquiry about any other medication could be useful, so that the nurse can assess any effect such drugs may have on elimination. For a female patient, any relevant gynaecological or obstetric history should be noted.

The information from such a history cannot be viewed in isolation. There are other factors which make management of the incontinent patient so difficult. These might include the following:

1   The patient is over 65 years old.

2   The existence of a concurrent illness.

3   The patient is unable to walk.

4   He has dependency in the areas of bathing and eating.

5   Speech pathology is present.

6   He is unable to perform a sequence of three verbal commands (Adams et al. 1966).

Satisfactory nursing management will also depend on an understanding of the normal physiological and psychological mechanisms that affect micturition and defaecation, and how these may become disrupted.

Micturition

Physical and psycho-social factors

The act of micturition, or passing of urine, results from a complex neurological interaction which, although basically the same for all human beings, once disrupted can present a different clinical picture between individuals. Even among stroke victims the pattern of urinary incontinence is rarely the same between two patients.

The bladder   At its most simple level, the bladder has a dual function: first, to dilate passively and contain the urine entering from the ureters until a certain volume and pressure are reached; and then, under normal voluntary control, to actively expel its contents in a socially acceptable time and place

(Stanton 1977). Urine will remain in the bladder as long as the intravesical pressure does not exceed the urethral resistance (Shuttleworth 1970). In this statement lies the essential guide to the understanding and, therefore, the management of the problem, when the balance is involuntarily upset.

The bladder is composed of smooth muscle (the detrusor) and traditionally it is described as having three layers, namely an outer longitudinal, a middle circular and an inner longitudinal layer. However, recent studies show that only at the outlet of the bladder are these individual layers preserved (Stanton 1977). The inner longitudinal layer is composed of widely separated muscle bundles, which are arranged in a radial fashion as they converge on the bladder neck. They continue into the urethra where they form its inner longitudinal layer. In addition, the second, outer layer of the urethra is derived from the outer coat of the detrusor. Therefore, there is no separate internal muscular sphincter at the exit of the bladder, as some textbooks claim; there is only an external urinary sphincter muscle (Tanaghoe and Smith 1966). However, some fibres from the detrusor muscle are inserted into the trigone, the imaginary triangle formed at the base of the bladder by the insertions of the two ureters, and the outlet of the urethra. This combination has been described as the base plate, the function of which is to allow the bladder muscle to exert a maximal closing effort on the proximal urethra, or bladder neck, thus providing an important contribution to the urethral sphincteric mechanism (Hutch 1972).

In normal micturition, the contraction of the detrusor muscle induces an opening of the bladder neck, and just before this occurs the pelvic floor muscles and the external sphincter muscle relax completely, allowing the evacuation of urine to take place.

Consequently, micturition can be defined as intravesical pressure overcoming outflow resistance. Under normal conditions, a simple rise in intravesical pressure does not result in incontinence. For example, when a cough or sneeze occurs, the intravesical pressure may be raised to the equivalent of 200 cm H_2O (water), but outflow resistance is not overcome, probably because the muscular arrangement described above allows this pressure increase to be transmitted equally to the urethra, so there will be no alteration in the pressure across the bladder neck (Shuttleworth 1970). The length of the urethra, which is much shorter in the female than the male, does not appear to be a contributive factor to incontinence. Incontinence will result only if the detrusor muscle power exceeds the outflow resistance, overpowering the voluntary contraction of the external sphincter muscle. This muscle cannot be relaxed voluntarily, and efforts to micturate will not produce a relaxation unless intravesical pressure is above the threshold value of 20-40 cm H_2O (Bell et al. 1972).

Nervous control   Nerve fibres from the bladder wall will give information about bladder fullness (Figure 5.1). The tension in the wall of the bladder will be proportional to the contained volume. Normally, sensations of bladder fullness will begin when about 150 ml of urine has accumulated. At 300 ml, the sensory fibres of the sympathetic nervous system begin to transmit feelings of discomfort, and at 600 ml extreme pain will be experienced, outflow resistance overcome, and involuntary incontinence occurs. This pattern may vary because of the rate of filling of the bladder, the presence of infection or loss of tone due to age.

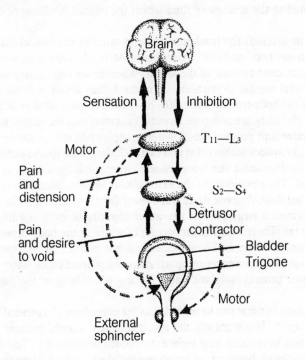

Figure 5.1 Innervation of the bladder

Although the reflexes of micturition can be activated in human beings through the spinal cord, the bladder and the external sphincter are normally influenced by centres in the forebrain. The cerebral cortex exerts an inhibitory control on voiding, which is modified by the afferent sensations of bladder distension and pain, and the knowledge that a socially convenient time and place exists. The stroke patient, especially one whose lesion encompasses parts of the frontal lobe, may have complex problems in micturition. Following a stroke there should be no particular abnormality of detrusor muscle power, or outflow resistance, so the act of micturition should continue to take place reflexly, even if the patient is unconscious.

Dehydration and thirst

The production of urine, and the consequent frequency of micturition, are directly related to the amount of fluid which the patient is willing or able to take.

We tend to overlook the fundamental importance of the role which water plays in both our body and our environment. After all, water is so abundant and familiar in most regions of the world. Whereas we can survive without food for several weeks, deprivation of water brings about a rapid death, usually after the body has lost up to 20% of its fluid content (Bell et al. 1972). The cells of the body are composed mostly of water, and are supported in a matrix of water and protein. Body water occupies two spaces in the body: intracellular, or spaces within cells; and extracellular, those spaces outside the cells. The latter includes the blood vessels, where it is spoken of as intravascular fluid. The remainder of the extracellular fluid is sometimes referred to as interstitial fluid. Adipose tissue has a lower fluid content than other types of tissue, because a large part of the water capacity of each cell has been displaced by fat. Therefore, the proportion of water in the body depends on the proportion of fat in it. So, the obese patient is more at risk from dehydration than his slimmer counterpart. Also, the proportion of water in the body decreases progressively with age, placing the elderly in the high-risk group.

The sensation of thirst can be regarded as the expression of a general bodily need for water. It is not merely the result of a dry mouth, because water deprivation produces thirst long before the mouth becomes dry. The neurophysiology of thirst, however, is by no means clear. Indeed, Epstein et al. (1973) claim that, while we traditionally think of just one thirst, there are probably four or five thirsts, which are as follows:

1   The thirst of cellular dehydration.

2   The thirst of hypovolaemia (blood loss).

3   The dry mouth, or prandial thirst (due to saliva loss).

4   Psychogenic thirst.

5   The drinking of palatable solutions, e.g. alcohol.

A patient with a dry mouth may not necessarily be dehydrated, and vice versa, but whatever the various sensory or internal environmental states in each case of thirst, all will normally lead to drinking behaviour. Elaborate mechanisms are involved for insuring the integrity of the circulation, by maintaining the volume and composition of intravascular fluid. In turn, the ability of the body to maintain homeostasis is particularly influenced by the excretion of, and lack of, water and sodium, two major constituents of extracellular fluid. Epstein et al. (1973) claim that multiple, overlapping factors are involved in control of water and sodium balances. For example, cellular dehydration, hypovolaemia, and the release of angiotensin, all stimulate the secretion of the antidiuretic hormone (ADH) during dehydration, and each appears to stimulate a desire for sodium in the diet as well.

Blass (1973) claims that only a 1-2% decrease in cellular volume is sufficient to stimulate the release of ADH, from the posterior part of the pituitary gland. Antidiuretic hormone acts directly on the distal tubules of the kidney, to conserve water, and causing the excretion of concentrated urine, resulting in a possible electrolyte imbalance.

Following a stroke, the patient is liable to develop hypernatraemia (high level of sodium in the blood), because of the effect of the cerebral lesions on such control mechanisms as are mentioned above, rather than a lack of fluid intake as such (Taylor 1962).

The water in the body is being continually lost and replenished. A healthy person, in a temperate climate, can maintain his water balance by drinking about 650 ml each day. He has, in addition, the water in his food, as well as that produced by the oxidative metabolism of carbohydrate, fat and protein (Bell et al. 1972). A minimum amount of urine, about 500-700 ml, must be passed each day, to allow the kidneys to eliminate the end product of protein metabolism (urea). This minimum quantity is increased if the patient consumes a large amount of salty food or protein. This should be taken into account when planning the nutritional management of the patient. Approximately 100 g of water are lost in the faeces each day, and about 500 ml is lost through the skin by evaporation, as insensible perspiration. Expired air, saturated with water vapour, accounts for a further loss of about 300 ml each day. All together about 4% of the total body water is lost in one day, but this loss is increased if the patient has a fever, is involved in excessive exercise or is breathing rapidly. Whatever the neurophysiological cause may be, the nurse should be able to recognize the symptoms of incipient dehydration in a patient. These might include the following:

1   Abnormal thirst.
2   Abnormal dryness of the skin and mucous membranes, with exceptional loss of elasticity in the skin.
3   A low urinary output (oliguria) with highly concentrated urine.
4   A confusional state.
5   The presence of fever.
6   Constipation.

Incontinence

Psycho-social factors

It is often difficult to differentiate between the physiological and psycho-social factors associated with incontinence. In stroke, for example, the level of awareness of the patient may not be separable from immobility as a reason for this disturbance. How many people, including nurses and doctors, remember when they last lost control, and were incontinent of urine and faeces? As the majority of nurses and medical staff are young and healthy, it is unlikely that many will be able to recall the difficulty they experienced when a child, or have experienced any difficulty associated with ill health. Unless they have endured being bedfast and reliant on others for elimination purposes, there is likely to be what Willington (1975) calls the 'experience gap', between the incontinent stroke victim and the nurse.

There will also be an 'experience shock' for the patient who loses control over urinary flow. Many find it difficult to express their feelings directly, because the process of elimination of waste matter is not normally referred to in polite society. Terms such as 'WC', 'the little room', or 'spend a penny', are used, or words which are not normally spoken before strangers (Dobson 1973).

Controlling micturition in a socially acceptable way also demands constructive, abstract thought. In our everyday life, we do not usually wait until our bladder is totally full before we retire to the toilet. To ensure freedom from discomfort and social embarrassment we anticipate any possible need, and 'go in case'. Misjudgment demands we seek a toilet in a public place, and this in turn demands mobility, and anticipation that we will be able to cope with any unknown obstacle, such as stairs. Most of the time we do not think too deeply about this process, but it demands an ability to plan for the future, i.e. to apply abstract thought. The stroke patient may have lost such an ability. He may not appreciate the appropriateness of using a receptacle before retiring to bed, or to avoid soiling his clothing, because he cannot construct the same mental image of the future situation as the nurse or relative. While the majority of incontinent patients will feel distress at their predicament, others may lack any interest in its social consequences.

The attitude of the patient is all important. Unless he can maintain a positive approach to the problem of regaining control, the nurse and family will face an uphill struggle. The nurse has a great influence on the patient's approach. Stockwell (1972), for example, claims that a nurse often uses sarcasm to promote what she considers to be desirable behaviour in the patient. Ridicule only increases the pressure on the patient, shatters his feeling of worth, and demoralizes him further if he believes he cannot reach the nurse's targets. Resentment is understandably generated if the patient shows a lack of interest in his lack of control, or adopts an aggressive attitude, using his incontinence as a 'punishment' of the carer, from feelings of fallibility. The nurse cannot help the patient if she does not seek to understand the reasons for his behaviour.

Equally unsuccessful is the nurse who takes a passive attitude to the patient's incontinence, an attitude that nothing can be done. The child-like position that the patient is driven to adopt in such a relationship can reinforce the incontinent state. Whatever the circumstances, some self-incrimination in the patient is almost inevitable, and he may retreat from reality as his self-image is threatened. Adequate stimulation, therefore, should accompany all retraining programmes. The nurse should not assume that simply placing an elderly patient among other elderly patients will benefit the incontinent. Studies show that incontinent persons, particularly the incontinent elderly, are extruded and ostracized from the company of all age groups, including their peers. This extrusion is maintained even after the individual has regained continence (Lipman 1968). So the elderly are no more supportive of the incontinent person than any other group, and cannot be expected to act with sympathy. So the nurse should not be surprised if she has difficulty persuading relatives, community staff, neighbours or volunteers to assist with the social rehabilitation of a patient, even when he has regained control. Suspicions that the problem may recur can erect defensive barriers, which the nurse or doctor may interpret as stubborn obstructiveness.

Researchers find that the disability of incontinence is not mentioned by sufferers, as other physical disabilities might be (Dobson 1973). Attempts may even be made, by the sufferer or spouse, to conceal the problem, or they may deny that it is a problem (Thomas et al. 1980). The patient's previous occupation and status may reflect the importance which control holds for him, and this may explain his level of anxiety. As Elhart et al. (1978) point out, psychic states of fear, cerebral excitement and embarrassment, increase the tonicity of the bladder muscles, and the stimulation to void becomes more frequent. Stress also increases the blood pressure of the body, which will in turn alter the glomerular filtration rate of the nephron, and reduce the reabsorption rate, resulting in a probable increase in the volume of urine produced. In addition, the stress of simply being in hospital can sometimes lead to a general diminution of interest in personal hygiene (McMillan 1966).

The complicated interplay between psychological and physical factors is well illustrated when a patient develops a conditioned reflex disturbance. Work on conditioned reflexes by Pavlov and others is well documented elsewhere, and will not be repeated here. In this process, elderly patients generally, and stroke patients particularly, often wet or soil themselves soon after they have been offered a bedpan, or have been taken to the toilet without success. The frustration which this arouses in the carer can often erupt in anger, because she mistakenly feels it was deliberate. Willington (1975) claims that if the psychological trauma is severe enough, the positive stimuli to eliminate (e.g. pressure on the buttocks by the bedpan) and the negative stimuli (e.g. clean bed clothing) become reversed. He calls this 'ultra paradoxical inhibition'. If it occurs, only careful assessment and planning will restore continence, and avoid the secondary reinforcement, which episodes of incontinence might offer.

Lack of urinary control has additional social consequences for the patient. The problem may be so severe that the stroke patient is afraid to leave his home. In addition, he may have to alter some social habits, such as alcohol consumption, e.g. drinking spirits instead of beer so as to keep down the fluid intake. Holidays and travel might be impeded. For example, public toilets tend to demand, especially for women, a coin in the slot, and have a strong spring on the door, while others have a heavy revolving gate at the entrance and exit. All such obstacles are difficult for the stroke patient to manipulate to gain access. The result may be that the patient drastically cuts down his outings, and may be made to feel a 'spoil-sport'. Single-sex public toilets prevent the husband helping the wife, and vice versa.

Financial complications may include extra laundry services and the cost of disinfectants and deodorants to combat odour. Furniture and floor coverings may be spoiled and have to be replaced, although those patients on supplementary benefits may be able to obtain a grant towards their replacement. Exceptional needs payments may also be available for replacing bed linen.

Assessing the patient's ability to micturate

Nordmark and Rohweder (1975) claim that the urinary output of any patient should be evaluated in relation to the following:

1 The quantity of urine the kidneys normally excrete within a period of time.
2 The total fluid intake.
3 The state of hydration.
4 Amount of fluid lost by other routes.
5 The emotional state of the patient.
6 The frequency and volume of each urinary elimination.
7 The main medical diagnosis, and related pathology.
8 Any diuretic drugs the patient may be receiving.

For the patient who is having difficulty with voiding, or who is incontinent, there are several additional factors which should come into the assessment, the accuracy of which will depend on the number and experience of staff available. These features are as follows:

1 The nature of the urine — whether or not it contains deposits, or has an abnormal smell, which might indicate infection or renal disease.
2 Incontinence specifications. These should include any relevant previous history, such as constipation or vaginal discharges. The time and quantity of the incontinence episodes should be charted, to indicate any trends in the situation.
3 A behavioural analysis. The patient's emotional reaction to the incon-

tinence episode is a vital observation. Also recorded should be whether or not the patient requested a receptacle, and if he was incontinent after attempting to use it. The period between evacuations should be noted, as well as any lapses of memory or inattention associated with micturition (Clipper 1975). Also relevant is whether he is incontinent in bizarre or socially unacceptable places.

If the patient can ask for, and use correctly, the receptacle, his conditional reflex mechanism is intact, and the prognosis should be good. If he asks for it, and then uses it incorrectly, the totality of the concept may have been lost. Table 6 shows how the nurse can test the extent of the patient's understanding of the elimination process (Willington 1975).

Table 6 Tests which can be used for assessing post hemiplegic incontinence (Willington 1975)

Sign	Disability	Special disability in elimination	Test
Dyspraxia	Inability to perform familiar activities	Inability to remember totality of voluntary muscular action for evacuation of bowel and bladder	1 Ask the patient to push down on the bowel, to produce a visible bulging of the perineum and anus 2 Ask the patient to relax and try to pass urine
Dysgnosia	Inability to recognize or to use familiar articles	Inability to recognize commode or urinal, or to position himself on them	Test his recognition of sanitary articles, and ask him to demonstrate how he would use them
Body image	Loss of cortical concept of body	Inability to clean genitalia	Ask patient to touch affected buttock with unaffected hand

When enquiring about success in recovery from incontinence, it is important to be sure that 'dry' nights or days are really the result of improvement in
the patient's control, and not simply a tribute to good nursing care. Persistent
incontinence in the absence of local causes is a discouraging prognostic sign.
Incontinence which resolves by 2-3 weeks after the stroke is more encouraging
(Adams 1974).

Defaecation and constipation

Constipation in a stroke patient is not a sequel to immobility as such, nor does
stroke always cause intestinal paralysis. Normal frequency of bowel movement depends upon several factors, including softness of stool, muscular
ability and control, and the heeding of the urge to defaecate (Mitchell 1977).
Whatever the cause of constipation, the management of bowel function
becomes extremely important for the rehabilitation of the stroke patient
(Hirschberg et al. 1976).

Physical and psycho-social factors

A study by Connell et al. (1965) found that 99% of their subjects had a bowel
frequency within the range of three bowel movements per week to three per
day. So while normal patterns of excretory function are variable, well-defined
limits to normality do exist. Factors which interfere with normal bowel habits
include the following:

1 Emotionally charged and stressful situations.
2 Limited mobility.
3 Embarrassment.
4 Depression.
5 Use of medications.

Illness, hospitalization or important occasions, which all promote stress and
anxiety, may disrupt normal bowel function, causing an increase in the
frequency of bowel movements. Long periods of confinement or travel, with
lack of exercise, tend to slow bowel activity or demand suppression of the
sensation to defaecate, with a resulting constipation. Simple exercises, such as
walking, normally necessary to maintain tone in the abdominal muscles which
are used in defaecation, may be denied the stroke patient for several weeks.
Whether a patient is ambulant or chairbound, any architectural barrier to the

toilet may be a critical factor which precipitates the onset of constipation (Nichols 1971).

Defaecation refers to the expulsion of faecal matter from the rectum. It is a complex act with both involuntary and voluntary phases, and requires the appropriate internal and environmental cues, and the appreciation of both. It involves not only the contraction of the rectum, with relaxation of both internal and external sphincter muscles, but also contraction of the abdominal muscles, including the diaphragm. During violent efforts at defaecation, the pressure in the rectum may rise as high as 200 mm Hg (Bell et al. 1972). Such a high intra-abdominal pressure can affect the return of venous blood from the lower body to the heart and, consequently, the blood pressure of the patient.

Faeces are moved along the intestinal tract by peristaltic movements of the muscular wall. Such movements are particularly pronounced after meals, or the drinking of hot or cold fluids. This is called the gastro-colic reflex, but its activity will be diminished if excitatory simultaneous stimuli, such as pain or noise, occur. The greater part of the intestinal tract demonstrates a large degree of autonomy, independent of nervous control from the cortex or spinal cord. Only the sigmoid colon and rectum are under the direct control of the nervous system. Some authors, for example Hirschberg et al. (1976), claim that a severe stroke can cause changes in the nerve supply to the rectum. It may be difficult, however, to separate such organic causes of constipation from more functional ones such as immobility or lack of awareness of the need to defaecate.

The rectum is normally empty until faeces are moved into it by involuntary action. The circular muscle fibres in the rectal wall are distended, and nerve impulses pass into the spinal cord and continue along the sympathetic pathways, to the cortex of the brain. When these sensations rise to the conscious level, a voluntary decision is made to defaecate. Stimulation via the para-sympathetic nerve pathways release the inhibition of the external anal sphincter. Voluntary control of the abdominal and respiratory muscles, and positive environmental cues such as comfort and privacy, allow expulsion of faeces to take place. This action is helped by the levator ani muscle in the pelvic floor, which contracts, pulling the anal canal backwards and upwards, over the faecal mass. Vaginal obstruction in a female patient can interfere with this action. The build up of abdominal pressure also affects the outflow resistance to the bladder, and micturition often precedes or follows defaecation. The length of colon emptied at each evacuation varies considerably. At the extreme, purgatives in full dosages may cause the large intestine to empty completely. The brain is able to distinguish between flatus and faeces, probably because flatus produces less distension in the rectal wall.

If the act of defaecation is postponed, for whatever reason, the sensation of rectal fullness rapidly fades. Indeed, even when the rectum contains faeces there may be no sensation or urge to defaecate. As the faeces remain in the colon, more water is absorbed, and the stools become hard round masses. Therefore, constipation can be defined as the retention of faecal matter, unusual delay in excretion or unusual deviation from normal elimination habits. If this process is not interrupted, impaction will result, and involuntary evacuation of liquid stool around the impaction begins. Such continuous soiling can cause deep distress, and increases the laundry burden of the carer.

In a 24 hour period, 135 g of faeces are normally expelled, constituting 3-8% of total energy intake. The composition of faeces depends very little on the constituents of the diet, except that the amount of roughage eaten affects the speed at which the faeces move through the colon. The composition of faeces, in the absence of any diet, remains unaltered, although the amount will become diminished (Bell et al. 1972) (Table 7). This table demonstrates that faeces are produced in the gastro-intestinal tract, and are not simply un-absorbed residues of food. Drinking large amounts of fluid does not alter the wet weight of the faeces.

Table 7 Composition of normal faeces

	%
Water	65
Solid matter	
(a) nitrogen	5
(b) fats	15
(c) calcium and phosphate	15

Assessing the patient's ability to defaecate

The nursing assessment of the bowel habits of any patient should be based on the following:

1   The usual pattern for bowel evacuation, including time of day and frequency.

2   The amount and type of diet.

3   The state of fluid balance.

4   Indications of possible constipation (Nordmark and Rohweder 1975).

If constipation is present, the patient may complain of one or more of the following symptoms:

1   A headache, general malaise and lack of appetite.

2   Feelings of rectal fullness, abdominal discomfort, and cramping.

3   Distension of the abdomen.

4   Absence of bowel movement, or passing small amounts of dry, hard faeces, with small amounts of liquid stool.

A history of the patient's bowel habits is essential, because it is especially difficult to establish satisfactory habits in persons who have suffered from constipation for many years, or who used laxatives or enemas before their stroke. Self-prescribed laxatives are a common feature of affluent societies, but their use is not always admitted.

Following stroke, the colour, consistency, amount and odour of the stool should not change. Nevertheless, the nurse should examine the faeces to exclude other pathology which may cause a change in bowel habits. For example, cancer of the colon is the second most frequent cause of cancer in midddle-aged men and women. For an unconscious patient, a digital examination should be carried out every 3 days, whether or not a bowel evacuation has been noted, as impaction can occur relatively high up in the colon.

Nursing management of the incontinent patient

The nursing management of the patient, whether in hospital or at home, will require a framework for assisting him to maintain optimal excretory function. Such a framework should centre on positive stimuli, including the following:

1   Prompt response to the patient's request for assistance.

2   Use of the commode or toilet as soon as physically possible, to reduce dependency and embarrassment, and reduce physical discomfort and the effort required to overcome the abnormal position imposed by the bedpan.

3   Placing toilet tissue close to hand, for the patient who is able to cope, and so that he will not have to risk upsetting his balance to reach it.

4   Provision of a signal or call device, for assistance.

Willington (1975) claims that the overall aim of caring for an incontinent patient should include the following:

1   Separating the patient from his excreta.
    a.   The means selected should have no harmful complications such as infection or skin lesions.
    b.   Offensive odours should be absent or reduced.
2   The social independence of the patient.
    a.   The patient should eventually be able to manage by himself.
    b.   The patient should be able to manage without serious disorganization, e.g. undressing.
3   The selected method of retraining should have some therapeutic component for the patient.
    a.   It should keep him warm and dry.
    b.   It should not present an affront to his ego.

The framework ought to allow opportunities to improve the patient's dietary and fluid intake, and to decrease any dependency on laxatives. It should also promote hygiene, e.g. through encouraging the patient to wash his hands after excretion. The nursing care plan devolved from such a framework has to take into account the level of understanding of both patient and relatives, and hence may have to centre on priorities, falling short of what the nurse may consider desirable. Certain generalizations can apply. For example, the patient should receive at least 2 litres of fluid each day in food and drink, but intake is best restricted after 5pm to reduce the desire to micturate at night and the risk of incontinence. If an outing, or other social occasion is planned, fluid restriction for 4 hours before the event will help. If the fluid intake includes pure orange juice or prune juice, this will reduce the patient's need for laxatives. Another example of general care might be that all incontinent patients should have their buttocks and perineal area washed and thoroughly dried at least three times each day, and after each episode.

This is extremely time consuming, and the risk of complications, such as pressure sores, often results in the patient being catheterized.

Use of catheters

When the patient is unconscious the bladder will evacuate reflexly, when a certain intravesicular pressure is reached. Timing the episodes of incontinence may allow a urinal to be placed in position in anticipation of micturition, or external tubing might be used for a male patient. As no satisfactory external appliance is available for a female patient, bedwetting is more problematic in women than in men. The typical incontinence pad provided for the health services, to the specifications of government (DHSS 1969), is of limited value, because it is designed to prevent wetting of the bed clothing and fails to separate the excreta from the patient's skin. More effective, if more expensive, pads are available, which absorb urine while maintaining a barrier between the soiled portion and the patient's skin. The general ineffectiveness of incontinence pads in the care of the unconscious patient can be a factor in the decision to introduce a catheter. The decision to catheterize an incontinent patient may also be taken on the basis of the possibility of infection being the lesser evil compared with the probability of pressure sores (Lowthian 1970).

If catheterization is essential to the welfare of the patient, a disposable, silastic in-dwelling catheter should be used as it will cause a less sensitive reaction in the urethral lining than catheters made of other materials. In addition, it can remain in situ for up to 6 weeks, thereby reducing the risk of infection from repeated catheterization.

Although infection in the bladder of an adult may take a long time to reach the kidney, this may not be so in an elderly patient (Talbot et al. 1959). Any reluctance to catheterize should not be carried to extremes, because as Gray (1973) points out, incontinence managed without a catheter might also result in a urinary tract infection.

There is no consensus as to whether or not a catheter should be clamped off when the patient is unconscious, or allowed to drain freely into a bag attached to the bed. The argument for free, closed drainage is that any urinary stasis precipitates infection. The counter-argument claims that clamping and releasing the catheter every 2 hours will help to retain the muscle tone of the bladder wall. The use of spiggots, especially wooden ones, to close off the catheter, cannot be recommended, because if improperly handled they can provide a source of infection. Excess tubing should be secured to prevent drag, and the usual cleansing techniques adhered to.

Once the patient regains consciousness, the catheter should be clamped and released 2 hourly, and removed altogether as soon as possible, and a retraining programme introduced if necessary. A stroke patient should not be allowed to retain a catheter for social reasons, neither should it be left in situ for the convenience of staff, because it will interfere with the progress of the patient, and means he must continue to receive medical and nursing attention.

Anticholinergic drugs, which increase the capacity of the bladder by interrupting nerve impulses, are virtually useless in most cases of incontinence (Bolwell 1982). Electrical treatment, or faradism, which involves the application of an electrical stimulus to the perineum to re-educate the pelvic muscles, is of no value to the incontinent stroke patient, and should not be attempted.

Retraining the bladder for continence

Timing The bladder always has some urine in it, but the nurse will not be able to palpate the distending bladder until it extends over the pelvic brim. Unless the patient can communicate his need, the nurse will have to base her judgement of his bladder capacity on palpations, and the length of time between episodes of incontinence. This information is important because retraining should start with the basic stimulus, the nearly full bladder. There is no point placing the patient on the toilet at a time to suit the nurse or relative, if intravesicular pressure is insufficient to overcome outflow resistance, however hard the patient tries. Neither will the patient be able to urinate unless he is in a relaxed state, both mentally and physically. Consequently, timing is critical, and leaving the patient on the toilet or commode when he has no urge to use it will make him uncomfortable, and anxious that he is not fulfilling the expectations of others, both of which factors will act in turn as inhibitors to urinary flow. Other negative stimuli include lack of privacy, cold and dirty toilets or receptacles, wrong position and the interference of clothing. To avoid ultra paradoxical inhibition developing, positive or excitatory stimuli should always be promoted. As well as a full bladder, Willington (1975) claims that examples of these would include the correct position to use the receptacle, the absence of relevant clothing, warm and clean receptacles or toilets and absence of odours. In addition, the sound of running water may help to stimulate urinary flow.

All those participating in the retraining programme should be made aware of the deleterious impact which negative stimuli can have, whether such stimuli are directly or indirectly applied. An example of an indirect negative stimulus is when the patient is made to sit on an incontinence pad in a chair. Because the pad is often not large or absorbent enough, two pads are frequently used, which advertizes the patient's incontinence. This is prejudicial to the patient's self-respect, and can make him feel, 'it doesn't matter anyway' (Bolwell 1982).

Clothing and incontinence The choice of clothing is important because it also acts as an indirect stimulus. Gammell and Joyce (1966) claim that the design of clothing for hospital use is often unsuitable for the incontinent, because soiled garments frequently have to be removed over the face and hair of the female patient. Nightdresses should be made, or adapted, to open all the way down the back, and secured by Velcro fastenings. Alternatively, they should open all the way down the front, and be buttoned so as to secure an overlap. Even if a woman is incontinent she should always wear pants when out of bed (Clay 1978a).

For incontinent male patients, experience shows that a long skirt may be better than pyjama trousers, as it may not get so wet (Smith 1981). However, cultural norms may confine this innovation to home care. The male patient should never be left without pyjama trousers or other similar covering, either in bed or in a chair. Any covering blanket rarely ensures the dignity of the patient when he is sitting in a chair, unless it is wrapped securely around the lower body, and then it is likely to become soiled.

Relatives can offer many suggestions for simple improvisations when encouraged by staff to become involved in problem solving.

Retraining regimes Clay (1978b) claims that a vital part of bladder retraining is for the nurse to gain the confidence of the patient by explaining to him, in simple but dignified terms, what is wanted of him. Whenever possible one nurse or relative should take responsibility. Having a different nurse or third person present may be embarrassing for the patient, and prevent him voiding. The atmosphere should be relaxed, for the patient may become agitated if he feels the carer is in a hurry.

A simple daily routine should be introduced, with success being reinforced by intermittent praise. Any mistakes or inattention should not be reproached. At 2 hourly intervals the patient should be asked if he wishes to use a receptacle, but he should only use it if he indicates a need to do so, or the nurse can palpate the fundus of the bladder above the pelvic brim. The result should be charted, including the time and the estimated amount of urine passed, e.g. small, medium or large, unless a more accurate assessment is required for other clinical purposes. Any episodes of incontinence should be likewise charted, and in hospital these charts should never be left at the bottom of the patient's bed. After 24 hours of recording, the timing of the bladder checks should be altered as necessary, and be carried out more or less frequently, depending on the bladder capacity of the patient.

At home, a simple device may be set up to remind the patient, or relative, of the time. The buzz of an alarm or cooker clock may be suitable.During the night the procedure should follow the daytime pattern, except that the patient should only be disturbed and encouraged to void if he is found to be incontinent at a certain time. A visual, 2 hourly check for incontinence can be carried out by the night nurse, without unduly disturbing the patient. At home, an electrical device which emits an audible signal when in contact with dampness may be useful. Night sedation for the patient should be kept to a minimum. Success can be put at risk by lack of attention to simple factors, such as the position of the patient's bed in relation to the toilet or a public throughway, or the distance which the nurse has to cover to bring the commode. Social elements have also to be considered; e.g. visits by relatives and neighbours may have to be shortened or rescheduled, to avoid embarrassment. The timing of any retraining programme carried out at home should avoid the busy times of the family's day, such as meal-times or when the toilet is in greatest demand. If continence is not established in 2-3 weeks, a complete reassessment should be carried out, reviewing possible local or systemic causes.

Incontinence pants   For irredeemable incontinence, or for those patients undergoing rehabilitation but who have not yet fully regained continence, special pants with pads inserted between the legs are available. There are many different commercial brands which may be purchased for the patient, but the one chosen should separate the patient's skin from the excreta, promote independence and have a therapeutic component. Many of the cheaper brands fail to achieve one or more of such criteria (Elphick 1972, Willington 1973).

The nurse's assessment when providing pants should include the hip as well as the waist measurement of the patient. She should check that the elastic leg band of the pants fits snugly, to prevent any leakage of urine down the leg, but is not too tight. For the stroke patient the type purchased should have the pad insert at the front, so he can eventually change the pad himself, without having to pull the pants off altogether. He should not have to pull them on over his feet; they should fasten at the sides, similar to a nappy or diaper (Broad 1972). The pants should be made of a washable material, which will dry quickly. They should be washed daily, and should not be worn in bed at night. Pads are available which can absorb up to 400 ml of urine before discomfort develops, so that the patient need only change the pad about three to four times each day.

Disposal of soiled articles   In hospital, the problem of disposal is not usually of direct concern to nursing staff. In the home, however, the trend away from heating by open fire, and the building of high-rise flats with new forms of rubbish disposal, make the removal of soiled articles more problematic. Methods of disposal which may be available are as follows:

1   Burning. The home fire can be used, or in rural areas an incinerator may be provided.

2   Flushing down the toilet. The manufacturer's recommendations should be checked before this is attempted.

3   The use of polythene bags. The health visitor should normally be able to arrange a supply of bags to the home, to avoid additional expense to the family. These can be disposed of by:
   a.   Ordinary refuse collection. Wrapping the pads in newspaper might reduce unpleasant odours.
   b.   A special collection by the sanitary services, through a special request by the health department.
   c.   A special collection by the health services may be available in some areas of the country (Dobson 1973).

Laundry services   If constant laundering becomes a burden to those caring for a stroke victim at home, then the community nurse can approach the social service department for assistance. In many cases, help can be offered with ordinary as well as soiled laundry. Exceptional need grants can help pay for extra bed linen, and possibly for assistance with fuel bills resulting from the need for extra hot water. The chief carer may be eligible for the Constant Attendance allowance, which can offset any loss of earnings or additional expenditure.

Bowel retraining programmes

Retraining the patient towards good bowel habits should be less time-consuming than retraining for continence. A normal bowel routine can be established even for a confused or unconscious patient. For most patients normal bowel habits can be regained in a few weeks and, once achieved, the habit is likely to be retained.

Unlike the bladder retraining programme, the bowel retraining process begins with an *empty* rectum. Consequently, in the first instance, any hard faeces will have to be removed, perhaps by the use of an enema. Thereafter, enemas should not be necessary, or desirable because they cause a loss of potassium, which leads to further atony of bowel muscle (Granger et al. 1975). A phosphate retention enema should be used in preference to soap and water, because of the risk of toxification from the latter. Faecal incontinence can be prevented in most cases by careful nursing and a high-residue bran diet (Shuttleworth 1970), but when it occurs, the obstruction may have to be removed mechanically by digital insertion. If laxatives are required, lubricants such as liquid paraffin ought not to be used, because they interfere with the absorption of fat-soluble vitamins from the intestine. Cathartics, including anthracene compounds such as Senokot, are safer. Another safe laxative, which should be taken at bedtime and which is fairly easy for the stroke patient to take, is danthran (Dorbanex) liquid.

Whatever method is used to empty the rectum, a digital examination should be carried out, to ensure that it has been successful, before the next stage commences.

A time is set for defaecation, e.g. three times per week, so that a distinct and definable interval exists between evacuations. The timing should take into account the previous bowel habits of the patient. It is easier to control the situation if the patient is slightly constipated. Evacuation is then achieved by the use of suppositories. Most authors advocate the use of bisacodyl (Dulcolax) suppositories which act about half an hour after insertion. The action of glycerin suppositories is less predictable. Two suppositories should be inserted between the faeces and the rectal wall, about 30 minutes after the patient has had breakfast. He should then lie down in a left lateral, or supine, position, to aid retention. After approximately 30 minutes, or sooner if he requests it, he should be helped onto a commode or toilet, and encouraged to push gently downwards to increase intra-abdominal pressure. The commode should always be preferred to the bedpan when the patient's condition permits.

For an unconscious patient, a reflex evacuation should take place following the insertion of suppositories, and an incontinence pad can be left in situ to collect the faeces.

Any bowel retraining programme may not be successful if concurrent attention is not paid to the patient's diet, and if his mobility is not maintained.

References

Adams, G F (1974) Cerebral Vascular Disability and the Ageing Brain, Churchill Livingstone

Adams, M, Baron, M and Caston, M A (1966) Urinary incontinence in the acute phase of CVA, Nursing Research, 15: 100

Bell, G H, Davidson, J N and Emslie Smith, D (1972) A Textbook of Physiology, 8th edition, Churchill Livingstone

Blass, E M (1973) Cellular dehydration thirst, in A N Epstein, H R Kissileff, and E Stellan (Editors) The Neurophysiology of Thirst: New Findings and Advances in Concepts, J Wiley & Sons

Bolwell, J (1982) Dignity at all times, Nursing Mirror, 154(14): 51-54

Broad, J N (1972) Urinary incontinence — a new method of control, Nursing Times, 68: 1212

Brocklehurst, J C, Dillane, J B, Griffiths, L and Fry, J (1968) The prevalence and symptomatology of urinary infection in an aged population, Gerontologica Clinica, 10: 242-253

Clay, E C (1978a) Incontinence of urine, Nursing Mirror, 150: 14-16

Clay, E C (1978b) Incontinence of urine — a regime for training, Nursing Mirror, 150: 23-24

Clipper, M (1975) Nursing care of the stroke patient, in S Licht (Editor) Stroke and Its Rehabilitation, Licht

Connell, A M, Hilton, C, Irvine, G, Lennard-Jones, J E and Mislewicz, J J (1965) Variations of bowel habit in two population samples, British Medical Journal, 2: 1095-1099

DHSS (1969) Specifications for disposable incontinence underpads, no. TSSD/D/300.00., HMSO

Dobson, P (1973) Management of Incontinence in the Home — A Survey, Disabled Living Foundation

Elhart, D, Firisch, S C, Gragg, S H and Rees, O M (1978) Scientific Principles in Nursing, C V Mosby

Elphick, L (1972) Incontinence, Disabled Living Foundation

Epstein, A N, Kissileff, H R and Stellar, E (1973) The Neurophysiology of Thirst — New Findings and Advances in Concepts, J Wiley & Sons

Gammell, A and Joyce, F (1966) Problems of Clothing for the Sick and Disabled, Disabled Living Foundation

Gray, W M (1973) Functional inefficiency of the lower urinary tract, Physiotherapy, 59 (51): 140-141

Granger, C V, Greer, D S, Lister, E, Coulombe, J and O'Brien, E (1975) Measurement of outcomes of care for stroke patients, Stroke, 6: 34-41

Hamerin, E (1982) Attitudes of nursing staff in general medical wards towards activation of stroke patients, Journal of Advanced Nursing, 7: 33-42

Hirschberg, G G, Lewis, L and Vaughan, P (1976) Rehabilitation, J B Lippincott

Hutch, J A (1972) The Anatomy and Physiology of the Bladder, Trigone and Urethra, Appleton-Century-Crofts

Isaacs, B (1979) Water, water everywhere — it's time we stopped to think, Royal Society of Health Journal, 4: 155-165

Isaacs, B and Walkey, F A (1964) A survey of incontinence in elderly hospital patients, Gerontologica Clinica, 6: 367-376

Lipman, A (1968) A socio architectural view of life in three homes for old people, Gerontologica Clinica, 10: 88-101

Little, D and Carnevali, D (1976) Nursing Care Planning, 2nd edition, J B Lippincott

Lowthian, P T (1970) Bedsores — the missing link? Nursing Times, 46: 1454-1458

McMillan, D (1966) Senile breakdown in standards of personal and environmental cleanliness, British Medical Journal, 2: 1032

Mitchell, P H (Editor) (1977) Concepts Basic to Nursing, McGraw-Hill

Mulley, G (1978) Stroke — A Handbook for the Patient's Family, Chest Heart and Stroke Association

Nichols, P J R (1971) Rehabilitation of the Severely Disabled Management, Butterworths

Nordmark, M T and Rohweder, A W (1975) Scientific Foundations of Nursing, 3rd edition, J B Lippincott

Patrick, G (1973) Forgotten patients in the medical ward, Canadian Nurse, 68 (3): 27-31

Shuttleworth, K E D (1970) Incontinence, British Medical Journal, 4: 727-729

Stanton, S L (1977) Female Urinary Incontinence, Lloyd Luke

Stockwell, F (1972) The Unpopular Patient, Royal College of Nursing

Talbot, M S, Mahonery, E M and Joffee, S J (1959) The effects of prolonged urethral catheterization on normal renal structure and function, Journal of Urology, 81: 138

Tanaghoe, E and Smith, D (1966) The anatomy and function of the bladder neck, British Journal of Urology, 38: 54-71

Taylor, W H (1962) Hypernatraemia in cerebral disorders, Journal of Clinical Pathology, 15: 211-220

Thomas, T M, Plymat, K, Blannin, J and Meade, T W (1980) Prevalence of urinary incontinence, British Medical Journal, 281: 1243-1253

Willington, D F (1969) Problems in urinary incontinence in the aged, Gerontologica Clinica, 11: 330-356

Willington, D F (1973) Marsupial principle in maintenance of personal hygiene in urinary incontinence, British Medical Journal, 3: 626-628

Willington, D F (1975) Incontinence, Macmillan Journals

CHAPTER 6

NURSING MANAGEMENT OF PERSONAL HYGIENE

Introduction

The need to provide adequate skin care for the stroke patient is reflected in several published nursing care studies (e.g. Rodrigues 1976. Hodgson 1977, McLaren 1977, Williams 1979 and Callum 1980). However, there is a tendency in such care studies to relate somewhat superficially to the physical and psychological relevancy of integumentary care within the wider context of personal hygiene. While it is recognized that the development of a pressure sore is one of the most catastrophic outcomes of low standards on skin care, other factors of personal care should not be overlooked. Such factors will be discussed under the headings of care of the skin, and care of the hair and nails.

Care of the skin

Functions of the skin

The skin is a complex, specialized organ with a variety of functions, the major one being protection, in that it is the body's first line of defence. This factor underlies all nursing activity relating to personal hygiene, and to maintaining skin integrity.

The skin is rich in nerve receptors which help apprise the body of its external environment, through pressure, pain and temperature sensations (innes 1977). The skin is kept supple, and the barrier maintained, by the secretion of oil, or sebum, from sebaceous glands. Dry or cracked skin will not be an effective barrier to the pathogenic organisms in the environment. Dry skin actually reflects the loss of water from the skin, rather than a loss of skin oil. The acidity of perspiration is responsible for retarding the growth of most human pathogens, by maintaining a skin pH of 3-5 (Billings and Stokes 1982). Any increase in the production of sweat reduces the acidity and disinfectant properties of the skin. Temperature regulation is another important function. Heat can be lost through capillary vasodilation and the evaporation of perspiration. Reversal of this process conserves body heat. Obese individuals tend to have difficulty in regulating their body temperature, because fat is a poor conductor of heat. Excessive perspiration results in the loss of water, sodium and non-protein nitrogen, all of which affect the fluid volume and osmotic balance of the body.

As any individual grows older, the dryness and scaliness of their skin increases, and sebaceous gland activity decreases. Changes also occur in the fibrous connective tissue, with an accompanying reduction in subcutaneous fat. This results in a thinning of the skin and a decrease in its elasticity, so it becomes wrinkled and sags into the folds normally associated with ageing. Superficial veins become more prominent. Sweat glands atrophy and perspiration is diminished. Age spots (senile lentigo) appear, as changes in pigmentation of the skin take place, while skin capillaries become fragile and tear easily. Consequently, as one grows older, the skin loses its ability to function efficiently, unless it receives careful attention. For example, as one ages the skin becomes less tolerant to the application of soap and water, and a more oily substitute should be used.

Following a stroke, the ability of the skin to continue with its functions will not be impaired. Nevertheless, the destructive effect of the lesion on the central nervous system may override local efficiencies. For example, interference with the temperature-regulating centre of the brain can lead to a rise in body temperature, and consequent perspiratory reaction (diaphoresis). Paralysis of the affected side will diminish the patient's normal ability to respond to traumatic situations. Loss of sensory awareness will be another complicating factor. The patient will not be aware of touch, pain or temperature changes at the cortical level, and this may result in serious traumatic injury. Reflex activity will continue to be present, despite cortical damage, because it can operate through the spinal cord, independently of the higher centres. The limb may jerk away from potential danger, but the patient may not be aware of it doing so. Sustained pressure or other stimuli will overcome the reflex action, and defensive reaction will be lost. The stroke victim is at risk from excessive pressure, and heat or cold injury, on the hemiplegic side. In addition, other factors such as the presence of urinary incontinence and excessive perspiration will diminish the ability of the skin to maintain its integrity. The extent of risk can be ascertained through the nursing assessment of the patient.

Nursing assessment

The condition of the skin and mucous membranes should be evaluated in relation to the following factors:

1   The severity of the disability following stroke.
2   Any relevant secondary disorder.
3   The patient's general physical status.
4   The emotional status of the patient.
5   Any history of hypersensitivity.
6   The age of the patient.
7   Any relevant medication which has been prescribed.

Any nursing assessment of the patient's skin must be thorough, yet inobtrusive, and should not lessen the dignity of the patient. Comfort and privacy, for instance, should be assured. Adequate lighting is essential if a close examination of the skin is considered necessary. Assessments of the skin are usually conducted during the first bathing procedure, unless indications demand otherwise.

The nurse should note the colour of the skin, its pigmentation and any abnormality such as redness, pallor or cyanosis. Bruises, which are local discolourations caused by capillary bleeding into superficial tissues, should be described according to their location, size and colour. The extent of any bruising or similar marks may indicate the ability of the patient to avoid possible injury. The fullness, or turgor, of the skin should be examined next. Such fullness will depend on the amount of fluid supporting the cells of the skin. For example, when dehydrated skin is pinched, it does not return quickly to its original shape, as does normal skin. This should not be confused with the inelastic reactions of the skin in normal ageing. If the skin is healthy it should spring readily back to its original position when stretched. An overabundance of fluid in the skin will cause swelling, or oedema. When hand pressure is applied to such an area, the finger marks or 'pits' will remain when the pressure is removed.

The nurse should look for any abnormal break in the surface of the skin, such as scratches or lacerations. Particular attention should be paid to the bony prominences most exposed to the risk of pressure sores (Figure 6.1). An accurate record of the length, depth and position of any such injury will form the base-line against which further evaluations will be measured. The assessment of any sensory loss has been described earlier, but the patient may complain of other sensory abnormalities, such as itching or pruritis of the skin.

Finally, the general state of cleanliness of the skin should be assessed, and any body odour noted.

The assessment of the ability of the stroke patient to cope with personal hygiene should begin as soon as his clinical condition becomes stable. A simple explanation should be offered before each stage of the procedure begins. When the patient is able to sit upright, whether in bed or, preferably in a chair, and his level of awareness is sufficient to proceed safely, the nurse should carry out the assessment in the following manner.

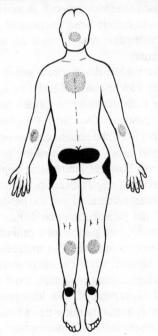

Figure 6.1 Pressure areas of the body associated with bedrest. The solid black areas are at immediate risk, while the dotted areas may become affected under certain conditions

A bed table of a suitable height should be placed over the bed or chair, to provide a secure base for the equipment. A plastic washbowl, with a large diameter, should be placed on the table in front of the patient, and liberally filled with warm, but not hot, water. He should not have to reach forward, or unduly alter his position, to reach the centre of the bowl, or the washing implements which have been provided. He should be well supported by pillows or other means on his affected side, because his tendency to fall towards that side increases the risk of an accident taking place.

After ensuring privacy, the nurse should approach the patient from his unaffected side and ask him to try to remove his upper clothing. She should note his response and offer help as required. The upper part of the trunk should then be covered by a towel, in case of intrusion and to ensure warmth. When she has gained the patient's attention, the nurse should instruct him in simple concrete terms about what to do next. For example, 'please wet your facecloth in the bowl of water'. From the patient's reaction she can assess his ability to understand the instruction, draw associations and perform the activity. It will also give the nurse information about the patient's conception of his altered body image. If there is no response to the instruction, it should be repeated a second time, in case the patient was merely being inattentive. If there is still no response, the nurse should demonstrate what is required, and then encourage the patient to copy the movement.

The rest of the washing procedure can be broken down into a series of simple, progressive activities, so an assessment can be made of each one in a similar manner. It would be useful to arrange these activities on a chart, so a record can be kept of the daily attempts of the patient. (A chart for washing the upper part of the body can be seen in Table 8). If the patient cannot proceed through these activities, the nurse should finish off the washing procedure, giving praise for what he has achieved, however limited this might have been. The assessment should be repeated next day and continued until satisfactory progress has been made, or it becomes recognized that the patient will make no further progress in this area. If the patient shows no difficulty pursuing the first activities, let him proceed at his own pace until a problem occurs, if at all. Simply leaving washing implements in front of an undressed patient, and suggesting he attempts to wash himself, while the nurse works elsewhere, has no therapeutic value. If the patient cannot remember what to do, or the nurse is not present to assess what he is capable of, then little progress will be made. In a busy ward, or when the community nurse has a heavy work load, the washing assessment should be rescheduled to a quieter time of the day. The time decided upon should, whenever possible, be adhered to each day.

The main problem for the hemiplegic patient, when washing the upper body, is attending to the unaffected arm, below the shoulder. The arm and hand can be washed by placing them in a bowl of water. Drying can be achieved by rubbing the arm against a rolled-up towel held between the knees and the weight of the hemiplegic arm.

Nursing management

Any disabled patient planning his daily washing routine needs access to hot water, but not necessarily a bath or wash basin (Nichols 1971). As regards washing cloths, several studies have been conducted by nurses in hospitals to ascertain the most cost-effective disposable material which can be used for washing the patient's skin. Cannon (1981) compared commercial items, such as Cellduk-t wipes, with paper towels and other absorbent materials, and claims that they are more effective and less wasteful cleaning agents (also Orr and Black 1982).

When a full bed bath is given to a helpless patient, in hospital or at home, two persons should always be involved, for the safety and welfare of the carers, as well as that of the patient. His inability to move and support himself will necessitate much rolling and lifting, and improper measures taken to achieve this will invariably cause unnecessary injury. As soon as the patient is confident in sitting, and able to wash the upper part of his body, bed bathing should be dispensed with, and the patient should be wheeled to the bathroom for hygiene purposes. At home, a wash bowl may have to be a substitute for a wash basin. The nurse should check that the wash basin is of a suitable height for the patient to sit up against and reach into without having to make awkward movements. If it is not suitable, the progress of the patient may be impeded by the frustration he feels from an inability to cope. Taking the patient to the bathroom should consume no more of the nurse's time than fetching and carrying water, but the therapeutic component will be valuable.

A call system should be available, or improvised, to give the patient a greater sense of security. A patient who feels he will be 'forgotten', once he is out of direct contact with the nurse for more than a moment, will be reluctant to use whatever facilities may be available, because of his sense of insecurity. At home various improvisations can be introduced to avoid carrying heavy jugs of water to and from the patient. For example, a length of hosepipe could be used, or a thermos flask to keep the water warm. However, because of the hazards of hot water, any such schemes should be given a practical trial before

Table 8 A chart for assessing the patient's ability to wash the upper part of his body

	Tick as appropriate				
	Carries out instruction			Does not understand instruction	Understands instructions but not associations
	1st time	2nd time	Demon-stration		
(All instructions should begin with the word 'please')					
1 Wet the cloth in the bowl of water.					
2 Rub some soap on the cloth.					
3 Wash your face and neck with the cloth.					
4 Rinse the cloth in the bowl of water.					
5 Wipe your face and neck with the cloth.					
6 Put down the cloth and pick up the towel.					
7 Wipe your face and neck with the towel.					
8 Place the towel under your affected arm.					
9 Wet and soap your cloth again.					
10 Wipe your affected arm with the cloth beginning at your *shoulder*.					

being adopted (Nichols 1971).

As soon as the patient's condition permits, he should be allowed to take a full bath or shower in the bathroom. Although this is not vital to good skin care, its refreshing effect will boost the morale of the patient. The nurse can find out through tactful questioning of the relative how frequently the patient usually baths at home. There are still many homes in Britain without a bathroom, and for many families the tin bath in front of the fire on a Friday night is still a reality.

	Tick as appropriate				
	Carries out instruction			Does not understand instruction	Understands instructions but not associations
	1st time	2nd time	Demon-stration		
11 Rinse the cloth in the bowl of water.					
12 Wipe your affected arm with the cloth beginning at your *hand*.					
13 Wipe your affected arm with the towel beginning at your *elbow*.					
14 Place the towel across your lap.					
15 Wet and soap your cloth again.					
16 Wipe your chest with the cloth.					
17 Rinse the cloth in the bowl of water.					
18 Wipe your chest with the cloth.					
19 Dry your chest with the towel.					
20 Place your unaffected arm in the bowl of water.					
21 Rub your affected arm against the towel.					
Well done!					

Before taking the patient to a bath, the nurse should be aware of how much water he usually uses, the preferred temperature of the water, and what position he normally adopts in the bath. His preferences, and his disabilities, may suggest that a shower rather than a bath should be offered. If a medi-bath is available, how it works must be explained to the patient beforehand. For someone who has not seen such a specialized bath before, a little encouragement might be required before he will use it with confidence. The bath, washing implements and clean clothing for the patient should all be got ready before he enters the bathroom. The use of a hoist has been discussed earlier.

The critical factor in the ability of the patient to progress in this area of self-care will be his confidence in his safety. A sense of safety can be promoted by having adequate numbers of carers present to support him, but not interfering with his efforts towards independence. The concern of the carers for the patient's welfare must be made obvious to him. Bathing in front of others is such an embarrassing occasion that a careless remark or attitude from a nurse can damage the ego and self-concept of the patient. The temptation facing the nurses or carers to talk amongst themselves should be avoided. Helpers should leave the bathroom as soon as they are no longer needed, and the bathroom door should be locked by the remaining nurse, to prevent intrusion. The status of personnel, or a task to be performed, does not constitute sufficient authority to violate the privacy of the patient without prior warning.

An anxious patient will be likely to want to cling to the side of the bath for support, and will be reluctant to let go to wash himself. If no other obstacle exists to his security, he should be allowed to cling, without being ridiculed, until his confidence builds up. If his confidence does not return, and he cannot be persuaded to wash himself, alternative means of washing should be resorted to, because prolonged failure in this area of care prevents progress in others.

To wash and dry the involved leg, the hemiplegic patient must be seated. He might find a bath seat is satisfactory or, if he needs more support, a sturdy plastic chair placed in the shower might be suitable. Alternatively, a plastic bucket filled with warm water should be placed in front of his chair, into which he can place the affected leg while sitting securely. If this method is used he should begin his washing activity with the lower part of the body first, and then wash the upper part at a wash basin.

After the bath or shower, the skin should be thoroughly dried. A large bath towel, made of cotton material, wrapped all around the patient, can absorb wetness without the patient expending energy. For more general washing, a large towel is difficult to manipulate unless hooked to the wall for support. Smaller towels should be available or, alternatively, a piece of roller towel with the ends fastened back, like mittens, may help.

A soap rack across the bath can be a hazard. One which hooks on to the side of the bath and can be removed should be used. The soap itself can be secured by a piece of strong string through the middle. Looping the string will allow the soap to be secured around the patient's neck.

A long-handled brush will help the patient wash his back, while a sponge rubber mop of similar length will help him to wash between his toes. A shower unit fitted to the bath taps might also help him to wash areas of the body which are difficult to reach. Whatever the patient's preferred method of washing, the perineal area should be washed and thoroughly dried at least once a day (Gibbs 1969).

The hemiplegic stroke patient should have no difficulty brushing his teeth with one hand. Soaking dentures in a suitable preparation will reduce the need for them to be cleaned, as brushing these will present some extra difficulty.

Shaving can be accomplished with one hand, using an electric razor. Many modern women use various methods to remove unwanted hair, including shaving. Returning growth can be embarrassing to women who are concerned about their appearance. The nurse should tactfully offer to help the patient remove any unwanted hair. Similarly, there are individual preferences in the use of deodorants, body perfume and facial make-up. When the patient uses make-up, she should be encouraged initially to apply it without assistance, because errors may indicate discrepancies in the body image of the woman. If she has any difficulty, the nurse should then intervene to complete the make-up. Lorenze and Cancro (1962) suggest that a positive relation exists between severity of dysfunction of visual perception and dressing and grooming failure.

Prevention of pressure sores

The use of a rating scale will help to determine the patient's potentiality for developing a pressure sore. Space permits only one such formula to be mentioned (Table 9). By assessing the status of the patient in each category, an overall score can be obtained. In the rating scale of Gosnell (1973), the lower the overall score assigned, the higher will be the risk that the patient will develop a pressure sore.

Pressure sores mean pain and discomfort for the patient, interfere with his rehabilitation, and consume valuable nursing time and other resources. In addition, the morale of the patient will suffer, because pressure sores are not socially acceptable, in that they are associated with uncleanliness. Barton (1977) estimates that there will be 30 000 patients with pressure sores at any one time, and that the greatest number of these are to be found in the most technologically advanced hospital wards.

Table 9 A rating scale to assess the risk of a patient developing a pressure sore (Gosnell 1973)

Score	Mental status	Score	Continence	Score	Mobility
5	Alert	4	Fully controlled	4	Full
4	Apathetic	3	Usually controlled	3	Slightly limited
3	Confused	2	Minimally controlled	2	Very limited
2	Stuporous	1	Absence of control	1	Immobile
1	Unconscious				

Score	Activity	Score	Nutrition
4	Ambulatory	3	Good
3	Walks with assistance	2	Fair
		1	Bad
2	Chairfast		
1	Bedfast		

To prevent breakdown of the skin, the position of the patient must be altered at least every 2 hours, or as frequently as necessary (Berni 1972). An area of skin should not be allowed to remain reddened for more than 10 minutes. No substance should be applied or rubbed into the skin that does not have a proven therapeutic value. Various aids and equipment are available to assist the nurse or relative to prevent pressure sores developing, e.g. sheepskins, which have been discussed on page 67. A Ripple mattress can be useful, especially if the patient is emaciated, because it provides a constant alteration of pressure over the areas of the body which are in contact with its surface. The main disadvantage of such a mattress is the noise of the motor, which can disturb other patients. There is also the risk that staff will reduce the number of visual checks on the patient's skin, from a sense of false security.

Most nurses develop their own preferences, and indeed prejudices, for various aids and equipment to assist in the prevention of pressure sores. It is not possible to discuss individual items here, but Dyson (1978) suggests certain criteria which can be adopted when such equipment is being assessed for possible use (Table 10).

Care of the hair and nails

Nursing assessment

As one grows older, changes occur in the hair and nails, as well as in the skin.

Table 10 Criteria for evaluating aids or equipment for use in preventing pressure sores (Dyson 1978)

1	Does the article work?
2	Is movement facilitated by the aid?
3	Can the aid spread the pressure of body weight so circulation is maintained?
4	Is ventilation of the skin possible?
5	How are the articles affected by incontinence?
6	How soon does the aid become ineffective with use?
7	Is the article comfortable and stable?
8	How heavy is the article, is it easily handled?
9	Will the product become a source of infection?
10	Is it more suitable for a sitting or recumbent position?
11	Is there likely to be any hypersensitivity to the material?
12	Is it easily washed and dried?
13	Is a lot of staff training required to use it effectively?
14	Is there a fire hazard?
15	Does it increase the risk of thrombosis?

Hair follicles in the scalp decrease in size and number, so that growth is slowed and hair is lost, and characteristic baldness may develop. In other areas of the body hair growth may accelerate, particularly in the ears, nose and eyebrows where it tends to become coarse (Billings and Stokes 1982). The hair tends to become grey as the hair follicles lose their ability to produce pigment. The growth of the nails also slows, and they become more brittle, appear ridged and have a tendency to flake.

Any assessment of the hair and nails should include the following:

1 Condition of the hair.
    a. Colour, texture, amount and distribution in relation to age.
    b. The state of the hair, e.g. is it well groomed, permed etc?
    c. Are lice present?
    d. Is the patient using any oil or conditioner?

2 Routine for hair care.
    a. The patient's normal daily care routine.
    b. Does a female patient wear curlers, or anything to fasten the hair?
    c. Normal washing routine, e.g. is shampoo used?

3 Condition of the nails.
    a. What is the length, shape and configuration of the patient's nails?
    b. Is there any discolouration, caused by bruising (black), calcium loss

(white flecks) or fungal infection (yellow)?

c. Are the nails dirty, and can this be associated with occupation?

4 Routine for nail care.

   a. What is the patient's preferred method of cleaning?

   b. How does he usually cut or trim his nails?

   c. Does the female patient use nail varnish or false nails?

For a hemiplegic stroke patient an assessment should also include his ability to brush, comb and wash his hair, and file or cut his nails. Such abilities will depend on intellectual as well as physical loss. An assessment procedure should be constructed similar to that described for washing, i.e. with definable stages, and concrete instructions given to the patient.

Nursing management

Hair An elaborate hair-style, such as one demanding many clips, will not be suitable for one-handed grooming. If the patient has long hair, plaiting might provide a comfortable style, but the plaits must be undone and brushed thoroughly at least once a day. Plaiting also needs the help of a friendly hand. Realism must be tactfully weighed against vanity.

When a person is bedfast, the routine daily care of the hair consists of brushing and combing as frequently as necessary, to distribute the oil along the shaft of the hair, and to prevent matting and tangling which occurs rapidly when the head is in frequent contact with the pillow (Innes 1977).

Other hair-care processes depend on individual choice. The frequency of washing, and the use and type of shampoo used, have as much to do with psychological factors as they have with physical ones. Most men are content simply to wash their hair as a part of their shower or bath, but women tend to be more fastidious. Coloured patients with thick textured hair may present additional problems. In addition, the application of certain oils to the hair may have some cultural significance other than to simply combat dryness. When cultural differences appear, the family of the patient can offer advice, and obtain the necessary large-toothed comb or oils. The use of a wig or toupet is an individual choice, but it should not be used as a substitute for normal hair care. A hairdresser may be able to give advice on individual hair problems.

Nails Care of the patient's nails involves cleaning and trimming to maintain a safe length and shape. For the hemiplegic patient, this presents mechanical difficulties. These might be overcome by fixing a metal nail file into a wooden handle, which can be held between the knees, and the nail growth on the unaffected hand will be controlled by moving them over the surface of the file. Similarly, a nail brush can be attached to the side of the wash basin by suction pads, and the patient is asked to move his finger ends back and forth across the bristles. Varnishing of nails demands greater skill and the patient may have to have the help of a friend.

When the patient has suffered sensory loss his efforts at nail care should be supervised until there is no risk of injury to his finger ends. Thick, hard nails are better cut after being soaked in warm water, or oil solution. Special nail clippers may be safer and easier to use than ordinary scissors. The services of a chiropodist should not normally be required, unless some other complication is present, such as an ingrowing toe nail.

References

Barton, A A (1977) Prevention of pressure sores, Nursing Times, 73: 1593-1595

Berni, R (1972) Stroke patient rehabilitation — a new approach, Journal of Practical Nursing, 22: 18-20

Billings, D M and Stokes, L G (1982) Medical-Surgical Nursing — Common Health Problems of Adults and Children Across the Life-span, C V Mosby

Callum, C (1980) A patient after cerebrovascular accident, Nursing Times, 76: 1961-1964

Cannon, J (1981) A disposable flannel and wipe for incontinent patients, Nursing Times, 77: 165-168

Dyson, R (1978) Bed sores — the injuries hospital staff inflict on patients, Nursing Mirror, 151: 30-32

Gibbs, G (1969) Perineal care of the incapacitated patient, American Journal of Nursing, 69: 124-125

Gosnell, D (1973) An assessment tool to identify pressure sores, Nursing Research 22: 53-59

Hodgson, S J (1977) A patient after cerebralvascular accident, Nursing Times, 73: 524-525

Innes, B (1977) Integumentary status, in P Mitchell (Editor), Concepts Basic to Nursing, 2nd edition, McGraw-Hill

Lorenze, E J and Cancro, R (1962) Dysfunction in visual perception with hemiplegia — its relation to activities of daily living, Archives of Physical Medicine and Rehabilitation, 43: 514-517

McLaren, M (1977) Come on, Jiminy Cricket! Nursing Times, 73: 1433-1435

Nichols, P J R (1971) Rehabilitation of the Severely Disabled, 2 — Management, Butterworths

Orr, J and Black, E (1982) A boost to morale, Nursing Mirror, 155 (2): 36-41

Rodrigues, A (1976) Cerebrovascular accident, Nursing Times, 72: 1838-1840

Williams, L J (1979) Rehabilitation of a patient after cerebrovascular accident, Nursing Times, 75: 1528-1530

CHAPTER 7

NURSING MANAGEMENT OF SLEEP AND REST

Introduction

Sleep has been described in many ways and from various angles; the scientist sees it as a biological phase or process, the psychologist as an important part in the stability of behaviour, and the poet in terms of awe and mystery. Cicero, for example, called it, 'the image of death', while Pope wrote of sleep and death, as 'two twins of winged rage, of matchless swiftness, but of silent pace'.

Sleep has been defined as, 'a state of inertia and unresponsiveness' (Oswald 1980). It can be differentiated from unconsciousness by the arousal of the individual to wakefulness, on application of sufficient stimulus. Kleitman (1967) takes the view that the natural state of the brain is one of resting, and that muscular activity and sensory bombardment are necessary to maintain wakefulness. Hayter (1980) claims that it is, 'a complex biological rhythm that is intricately related to other biological rhythms and body functions', e.g. body temperature and concentration of urine. Dement (1974) believes that the human being essentially sleeps during the hours when he is least efficient, i.e. during the depressed stage of circadian rhythmicity.

What are circadian rhythms?

The universe is not static. Since its beginning life has evolved in the context of a rhythmically varying physical environment. Day and night come and go, the tides rise and fall along the seashore, and the seasons change. Every living component from an individual electron to a whole galaxy is continually moving, and such movement cannot proceed forever in the same direction. Sooner or later it will complete a circle, or stop and return in the opposite direction; in either case, a continuously repeated rhythm, cycle or periodicity ensues.

Within an evolutionary framework the human organism developed autonomous rhythmic processes, the periods of which had a tendency to match those of the environmental process. Today, however, environmental periodicity no longer acts as the chief cause of biological rhythm, but acts rather as a synchronizing agent or, as Aschoff (1966) called it, a 'zeitgeber', or 'timegiver', for self-sustained oscillations within the body. There is probably no function or organ in the body which does not show rhythmicity to some degree, so the nurse should understand both the concept and effect when planning the care of the patient (Myco 1981). 'Zeitgeber' describes any agent or stimulus, either physico-chemical or social, which enables a synchronized activation of the multivariate circadian periodicities which form the construction of habitualized everyday existence. The introduction of a new 'zeitgeber', such as a change of lunch hour, disrupts routine, acts as a stress stimulus, and requires adaptation until the person feels comfortable within the new time scale, i.e. until symptoms of physical or psychological hunger decline.

Halberg (1953) introduced the term 'circadian', to describe the self-sustaining rhythms which cover a period of about a day (Latin circa = about, diem = day). Although such rhythms may 'free run' within their own frequency for months, they can be trained to respond to physico-chemical, as well as social 'zeitgebers', to alter the period of their rhythm.

Owing to the ascendancy of circadian rhythms, a person becomes a different biochemical, physical and psychological system at each hour of the day. Any stimulus, or stress, might therefore be expected to have a different effect, or evoke a different reaction, depending on the phase at which it encounters the individual's circadian map.

The modern social world contains rigid temporal programmes which act as cues to the person's own temporal organization. These clues include the cycle of daylight and darkness, with its geographical and seasonal variance, calendars, diaries and timepieces. With accelerating technological advances, work activity is no longer influenced by the events of dawn and dusk, but by the school, office, factory, home or hospital clock. Food and fluid intake, once stimulated by physiological signs of hunger and thirst, now tend to be a response to set hours of the day, and have become an integral part of social activity, regardless of physiological needs. As a result of adaptive cycles, each person becomes programmed, through his social world, to do the right thing at the right time. Sleep and rest periods are part of this adaptive process.

When someone enters hospital, the environmental programme of the agency offers cues, or 'zeitgebers', dramatically different from those previously known and adapted to, whether as a single cue or as a whole. During the first few days a resynchronization has to take place, if there is an alteration present between the patient's previous rhythms and the new environmental cues. For example, a night shift worker will resynchronize his usual nocturnal rhythms of sleep activity, or food and fluid intake, to daytime patterns, as the context of his illness allows. The more years he has been involved in his occupation, the longer such adaptation will take. Neither should the spouse of a shift worker be forgotten. For example, the wife of a farmer, or milk delivery man, will be used to rising very early to help her husband.

Perhaps the most dramatic circadian rhythm is the alteration between the consciousness of the waking hours, and the reduction of the conscious state through sleep. The amount of sleep we have in a single unit, within a 24 hour cycle, is influenced primarily by social and occupational pressures. Without these pressures, the sleep-wakefulness patterns would probably be polycyclic, i.e. contain multiple periods of small amounts of sleep, rather than one single period. We are all aware of periodic waxing and waning of sleepiness during the day. This can be observed particularly among the institutionalized elderly, who are not involved in diversional therapy. Daydreaming is a form of microsleep. Singer (1974) claims that daydreaming or inner fantasies and thoughts help maintain an interesting environment when a person is confronted by monotony.

Many influences maintain wakefulness, such as anxiety, a high sensory input or an interesting, active occupation, while we become sleepy through boredom, warmth, comfort and a limited sensory input. The decision to go to sleep. Singer (1974) claims that daydreaming or inner fantasies and thoughts rhythm, which imposes certain moments of maximum likelihood. A patient who develops a polycyclic sleep pattern, rather than keeping to a single unit pattern, is not necessarily at a disadvantage in meeting his rest requirements. He may be helping his recovery more than someone who has his sleep pattern imposed by hospital routine or medication.

The stages of sleep

The overall pattern of a typical 'good night's sleep' can be recorded on an electroencephalogram (EEG), which detects the minute electrical changes taking place in the brain. This pattern can be subdivided into distinctive stages.

When the eyes are first closed, the 'alpha' rhythm of relaxation is recorded. The brain is functioning in a state of vigilance, and this rhythm disappears if the eyes are opened, or the brain is stimulated into a higher level of alertness. As the patient becomes more relaxed and enters Stage I sleep, the alpha waves are superseded by small, irregular recordings. At this stage, which usually lasts only a few minutes, the muscles are still in a state of tonus, and as we sink into sleep, the 'myclonic jerk' or shudder may occur, and cause arousal from the drowsy state (Hartmann 1973).

Stage II is said to have been reached after about 10 minutes of light sleep. The patient would be unaware of his surroundings, but could easily be awakened. There is a hierarchy of diminishing sensory perceptions, with hearing the last sense perceived before falling asleep. The eyes begin to roll slowly and blindly from side to side, and the brain recordings are characterized by sharp bursts of regular waves lasting only 1 or 2 seconds.

Gradually, the patient enters Stage III sleep. Muscular relaxation occurs, respirations become regular, and heart rate, blood pressure and temperature recordings continue to fall. This has the effect of reducing the basal metabolic rate by 10-20%.

Finally, deep Stage IV sleep is reached. This is characterized by large, slow, so called 'delta' recordings on the EEG. Arousal is now difficult, and may take several seconds (Figure 7.1).

These four stages contribute what has been variously described as orthodox, classical, light or non-REM (rapid eye movement) sleep. Approximately 80% of sleep is spent in rapid descent and ascent through the different layers. After about 90 minutes of such sleep, there is a gradual return to a Stage I state. However, instead of wakening, the sleeper proceeds into REM-type sleep.

Rapid eye movement sleep is also known as deep or paradoxical sleep, for although the sleeper has surfaced to a state very much like that of waking up, he is far more difficult to arouse than at any other phase of sleep. This is

Figure 7.1 EEG tracings of the phases of sleep

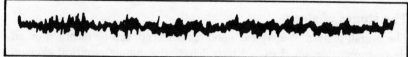

'Alpha' rhythm

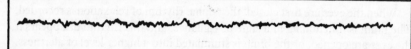

Stage I sleep — drowsiness

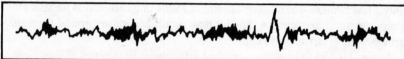

Stage II sleep

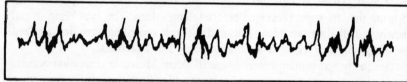

Stage III sleep

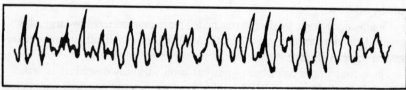

Stage IV — 'delta' sleep

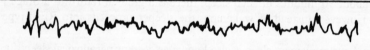

REM sleep

because he is withdrawn from reality, and prepared for action in his personal world of dreams. REM-type sleep is characterized by the imposition of saw-tooth waves on the EEG recording, with simultaneous eye movements and autonomic muscular twitching (Figure 7.2).

Figure 7.2 The progression of sleep stages in a normal night's sleep. Note how the first REM period occurs just over 1 hour after sleep onset; how the start of successive REM periods is bout 90 minutes apart; and how the length of REM periods builds up over the night, and the amount of slow-wave sleep, stages 3 and 4, declines.

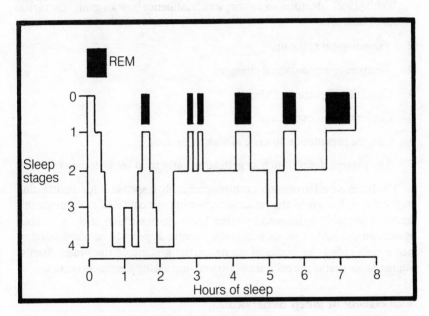

Each individual has an average of four to six cycles of sleep each night, each cycle lasting about 90 minutes, giving a total of 7-8 hours of sleep. However, cycles can range from 60-120 minutes, and they tend to lengthen with age (Webb 1968). Consequently, each patient needs a minimum of 90 minutes' uninterrupted sleep. Although the total sleep time is the same as for other adult age groups, elderly persons wake more often, stay awake longer, and may need to spend longer in bed to attain the same amount of sleep as others (Feinberg 1969). A polycyclic sleep pattern is more likely to impose itself on an elderly hospitalized or bedfast patient.

Within each sleep cycle, Stage IV sleep progressively decreases and REM-type sleep increases. Consequently, most Stage IV sleep occurs early in each night, and REM-type sleep during the few hours before wakening. The total amount of orthodox and paradoxical types of sleep varies. For example, REM-type sleep increases after unusually emotional days. Cycling of sleep also occurs during daytime naps. Morning naps are composed of large portions of REM-type sleep, while afternoon naps are proprtionately higher in orthodox sleep. Therefore, afternoon naps can be more easily reduced without loss of well-being to the patient.

Webb (1968) identifies six factors which influence how long any one person sleeps. These are:

1   Physiological make up.

2   Temporary physiological changes.

3   Conditioned pattern of sleep.

4   Current stress level.

5   Current presence or absence of task to be done.

6   Any present desires, such as getting up early for a pleasurable event.

The brain is said to contain a centre specifically responsible for maintaining wakefulness, known as the reticular activating system (RAS), although this centre is probably influenced by other brain centres which apply a braking system on the RAS. One such inhibitory centre appears to be a collection of nerve cells called the nuclei of raphe, at the midline of the brain. Animal studies show that if the cells are destroyed, increasing sleepiness occurs.

The effects of sleep deprivation

Sleep is commonly regarded as the great healer and restorer. To Shakespeare's Macbeth, sleep was 'sore labour's balm'. Adams (1979) claims that the main function of sleep is to be the stimulus to the restorative processes. Experiments in sleep deprivation have shown contradictory reactions in similar groups. However, after about 4 days of total sleep deprivation, healthy people begin to display a variety of physical and psychological symptoms. These include increasing fatigue, difficulty in concentration, episodes of disorientation and misperception, and general irritability (Johnson 1969). These symptoms tend to be more apparent in the early morning. According to Dement (1960), only in extreme cases will hallucinations develop, among susceptible individuals. For example, Dement (1974) gives an account of a man deprived of sleep for 200 hours who developed acute paranoid psychosis. Dement claims that hallucinations appear to be a breaking-through of much needed REM-type sleep into the waking psyche. Biochemical factors, e.g. corticosteroid levels, probably play a role in whether or not the symptoms of sleep deprivation develop. Sleep deprivation can be said to affect tissue renewal in the body. Tissue renewal appears to be stimulated during sleep through an increase in the synthesization of protein.

A patient who is deprived of sleep will become increasingly uneven in his level of performance of activities of daily living. He will develop weariness and apprehension, show lapses of attention, and have a tendency to become withdrawn. All unnecessary movement will stop, and the patient may begin to complain about unpleasant physical symptoms, such as headaches. With tiredness, changes in the perception of depth occur, and the outline of objects may appear blurred.

Adams (1979) claims that, by forcing us to sleep, the body clock ensures that the necessary repair work can be carried out, and at the most favourable time.

REM-type sleep is important, because it allows the nervous system to maintain a high level of activity, and thereby to practise skills before they are actually used in everyday living, like an actor learning his lines (Martin 1975). There is evidence that this dream stage of sleep plays a vital part in the problem-solving function of the brain. For example, after many years of searching for the answer to the structural riddle of the benzene molecule (C_6H_6), the German chemist Kekule is said to have had a dream in which he saw six snakes biting each other's tails and spinning round in a circle. When he awoke he interpreted the six snakes as a hexagon, the elusive structure of benzene. The old advice of 'sleep on it' is often worthwhile. Psychoanalytical theorists, such as Freud or Jung, claim that dreams allow us to settle unresolved conflicts repressed into our subconscious. By 'acting out' fears in our dreams, we can come to terms with them. Dreams, therefore, appear to be essential to mental health.

During REM-type sleep, the muscles of the body become totally flaccid and relaxed, although the brain is active.

Insomnia

Insomnia is a complaint, not a disease or illness. Most people assess their sleep inaccurately, usually exaggerating wakefulness. Dement (1974) claims there are two main categories of insomnia, namely ideopathic and pseudo-insomnia. Ideopathic insomniacs tend to be in the minority. They tend to have little sleep and are easily aroused, and there are disturbances in the sleep recordings of their EEG. The pseudo-insomniac claims never to have slept at all, despite appearing to sleep soundly, and with EEG recordings which confirm that state. These patients are not simply moaners, because there are physiological differences between those who wake feeling rested and refreshed, and those waking to a feeling of fatigue and lethargy. Such physiological symptoms are confirmed by brain-wave patterns, and heart and temperature recordings. Poor sleepers do not sleep so deeply, their body temperature does not decline so low at night, nor rise so early in the morning. They have a greater percentage of Stage II sleep, and correspondingly less REM-type sleep, with more body movements, a faster heart rate and greater peripheral vasoconstriction while asleep. Rentschafen and Monroe (1969) found that, when awakened from orthodox sleep, insomniacs frequently claimed they were not sleeping. Poor sleepers, therefore, have heightened systemic activity levels, and thus they fail to experience the restorative benefits of sleep.

Luce and Segal (1967), in a survey of good and poor sleepers, found certain psychological characteristics shared by poor sleepers. These subjects tended to be more anxious, introverted, hypochondriacal and emotionally disturbed than good sleepers. They concluded, 'people who generally sleep poorly are psychologically different from those who ordinarily sleep well'.

Even when any apparent problems are resolved, insomnia can persist, as sleeplessness tends to reinforce itself, and once a pattern of sleeplessness has become ingrained, it is difficult to alter (Tyrer 1978). The stroke patient is at risk from what have been described as 'obsessive ruminations'. These are conscious or real concerns that are not easily resolved, such as worries about adapting to paralysis, or thoughts and fears about death. Such dilemmas will cause sleeplessness by forcing themselves persistently into the patient's thoughts. If a stroke victim acquired his disability during sleep, he may be frightened to sleep in case he has a recurrence of such a traumatic experience. Some causes of insomnia are more easily discernible, such as pain, stimulants and situational factors. Stimulants before retiring are counterproductive to relaxation. Excessive exercise, drinking beverages high in caffeine, and eating certain foodstuffs should be avoided in the evening whenever possible. Pain is a primary cause of sleeplessness (Choi-Lao 1976). Stroke victims find that the discomfort of heavy hemiplegic limbs, or subluxation of the shoulder, often makes sleep impossible. Situational causes of insomnia usually include excessive noise, bright light, an uncomfortable bed and excess heat or cold.

Nursing assessment of sleep disorders

Some forms of discomfort, such as wetness or fatigue, may be relatively minor and simply annoying for the patient, while others, such as pain, may be so distressing as to exclude all other concerns. However, they will all detract from the patient's ability to rest and sleep.

While nurses firmly believe that sleep is a great restorer, it tends to be a view that is more a vague, personal feeling than anything else. Nurse education tends not to highlight the importance of sleep in the recovery of the patient; rather the emphasis tends to centre on active care and active attention to his needs. Sleep is often misinterpreted as a passive phase of care. This is reflected in the frequency of its disruption by nurses and other staff. Patrick (1973) found that nurses did not understand the stroke patient's need for rest and sleep, or how to balance bedrest with stimulation and mobility, such as getting the patient up in a chair. The nurse has the responsibility of observing the patient for signs of fatigue. This demands that she should confer with other members of the health care team, to arrange an activity schedule for the patient, which will provide adequate rest periods. Fatigue can, and will, hinder the patient's performance and ability to learn what he is being taught. Schultz (1973) quotes a case where compounded fatigue in a stroke victim, whose activity schedule was too intense, contributed to the patient developing bronchopneumonia from which she died. Even general ward activities not directly applied to the patient can introduce feelings of fatigue after a while.

In hospital, all patients, whatever their previous sleep history or current needs, tend to be encouraged to meet their rest needs in one single unit of sleep. For a stroke patient, a polycyclic pattern of sleep might prove more beneficial. Consequently, a sleep history and assessment becomes a vital nursing tool. A sleep history should include the following:

1   The number of hours he sleeps, and the timing of his sleep, e.g. 11 pm - 6 am.

2   His pre-retiring habits or ritual, i.e. is there any order for undressing, washing, shaving or reading?

3   What relevant situational factors apply, e.g. sleeps alone, dislikes light, prefers good ventilation, likes to have two pillows.

4   Any medications taken to promote sleep.

5   Any secondary condition which interferes with sleep, e.g. rheumatic pain.

6   The patient's subjective feelings about his normal sleep pattern.

This assessment will provide a framework against which sleep problems can be compared. It should be seen in the context of the overall welfare of the patient, because many of the changes which might occur in his mood or behaviour pattern may be nothing at all to do with his personality, or his stroke, but simply the result of not getting enough sleep.

Nursing management for the promotion of sleep

Environment

Many patients, on leaving hospital, complain of what Clark (1980) called the 'sound and light show'. This is the disturbance caused by the activities of nursing and medical staff in the ward at night. While no one resents the attention offered to seriously ill patients, Garner (1978) claims that the therapeutic value of sleep is unnecessarily denied many hospital patients.

Examples of night noise can be placed into three categories, namely external noises, staff noises and patient noises (Whitfield 1975). External noises include the telephone ringing, lights, buzzers, creaking beds, commodes being wheeled about, and other equipment noises such as the motors of ripple mattresses. Examples of staff noises would include squeaking shoes, talking, nurses' observations and treatment of ill patients. Finally, patient noises include coughing, sneezing, snoring, breaking wind and calling out.

The problem of light appears to be a major situational cause of sleep disturbance in hospital. Electric lights are not usually dimmed before 11 pm, yet patients retire to sleep some time before this. The misuse of a night flashlight on nurse's rounds can not only disturb a patient, but confuse him because he can see little else while being blinded by the beam, on his sudden arousal.

The ventilation or temperature of the room should be adjusted to the patient's wishes whenever possible. A warm bed can promote relaxation; however any hot water bottles, or other form of heating, should be removed or switched off before the patient gets into the bed.

Continuous hourly checks on patients compound the mental stress of illness by interrupting sleep cycles, leading to restlessness and confusional states (Hilton 1976).

Patient

As far as possible, the patient's bed or rest time should be flexible, and organized to suit his wishes, and not for the convenience of others. This is easier to achieve at home than in hospital, but modern hospital wards give more scope to the planning of rest than do the older Florence Nightingale type of ward.

The stroke patient, because he suffers fatigue so readily, will want to rest during the day. Movement from bed to chair demands time and physical effort from the carer, but leaving a stroke patient immobilized in a chair, ignoring his pleas to return to bed, has no therapeutic value, although some nurses will present it as such. It is not too harsh to say that the discomfort and complications which such lack of care is fostering are so severe as to border on criminal neglect. Just as untherapeutic is putting a mentally alert, though physically disabled, person routinely to bed, from teatime until after breakfast next day. They are likely to fall asleep in the early evening, out of boredom and, having completed their natural span of sleep, wake up in the early hours of the morning, often disturbing other patients. Starting the patient's night at five in the evening decreases his opportunities for social activity which would stimulate a need for concentration and mental alertness.

While little can be done to promote the comfort of the hospital bed, relatives of the patient may wish to bring his top pillow or other articles from home, which encourage sleep. The patient should be allowed to wear his own night clothing as soon as possible. The act of dressing and undressing is a stimulus to wakefulness and sleep, so these activities should be included in his rehabilitation programme as soon as his condition is stable.

The waking time of patients should also be flexible. At home, this will have to fit in with the rising schedules of other family members. If the patient has to wake early, whether at home or in hospital, he should be allowed a morning nap, to ensure he is receiving adequate amounts of REM-type sleep. Paradoxically, hospital care centres on high activity levels in the morning, and if the patient is allowed a nap, it is usually in the afternoon, when REM-type sleep is unlikely to occur. The stroke patient in hospital should never be disturbed simply to have his temperature taken.

Exercise is conducive to sleep, both to the total amount and to the promotion of the deeper stages of sleep. However, strenuous activity should not be carried out within 2 hours of the patient retiring. Listening to music, talking or reading may promote the urge to sleep. The traditional warm milk drink has proven scientific value for sleep promotion. Milk, like other proteins, contains the amino acid L-tryptophan, which is a precursor of the neurotransmitter serotonin, which is believed to promote sleep through its action on the nuclei of raphe (Jouvet 1969). The amount of other fluids should be restricted in the evening to decrease the desire to urinate after the patient has retired. The awareness of a full bladder and fear of incontinence will interfere with sleep. A warm bath and a massage promotes relaxation and reduces mental tension. Alcohol in excessive quantities reduces the amount of REM-type sleep which the drinker has, although a drink at bedtime may help the patient to relax.

Settling the patient for the night is worth more than any sedative (Hopkins 1980).

Sedatives

Hypnotic drugs should only be given to the patient as a last resort. Taking such drugs every night reduces their potency, and dosages have to be increased to obtain the same effect. Consequently, the nurse should suggest that they are taken only when absolutely necessary, to avoid tolerance to the drug building up. They should be used only as a part of the patient's overall treatment and activity schedule; otherwise they can promote confusion, and induce hangover effects which interfere with the patient's performance.

In a study of the use of sleep medication, Gillies (1976) claims that when the nurse failed to determine the reason for his inability to sleep, the patient did not experience relief from sleeplessness even when medication was given. This claim is supported by Zelechowski (1977), who believes that the best results in helping a patient to sleep are obtained through scheduling his care to suit his own preferences.

A behavioural state which resembles sleep can be brought about by a variety of drugs. Barbiturates are known to alter sleep. Drugs, such as quinalbarbitone (Seconal), quinalbarbitone/amylobarbitone in equal parts (Tuinal), and pentobarbitone (Nembutal), markedly reduce REM-type sleep, so their aid to effective sleep is somewhat self-defeating. Because the patient becomes so markedly dependent on increased dosages, barbiturates are rarely prescribed in Britain today.

Idiosyncratic reactions to sedatives result in trial-and-error prescribing, as the doctor tries to find the right drug, in the right amount to meet the demands of the patient. The aim should be to find a drug which will bring about a rapid induction of sleep, has a short action and has no hangover effect, while maintaining as normal a sleep rhythm as possible. The literature contains several studies carried out to compare the effects of various agents. For example, chlordiazepoxide (Librium), which is frequently prescribed for stroke patients, is only effective as a sleep inducer for the first 3 days of administration. In a study by Hartmann and Cravens (1973), chlordiazepoxide was not inducing sleep (and was actually decreasing the amounts of deep sleep the patient had) only 3 weeks after the original prescription. In contrast, they found that chloral hydrate preparations did not disturb sleep patterns, and continued to be effective as a hypnotic 1 month after initial administration.

Whether or not hypnotic drugs are used, the nurse or relative must secure the safety of the patient at night. Within the wishes of the patient, the carer should see that he is properly supported by pillows, that the cotsides or a chair are in position, and that a night light is at hand if he requires it. If the patient is used to having a bedside clock, this should be retained, within easy reach of the patient's unaffected hand. Sometimes the rhythmic ticking of a clock is an aid to sleep. Sedatives should not be left on a bedside table in case of accidental overdose. Unless the patient is able to move easily, a urinal or commode should be on hand in the sleeping room. Many older houses still have outside lavatories, and the provision of a commode becomes essential under such circumstances. The administration of sedatives increases the risk that an accident may happen. Sedation should not be given during the hours of daylight. Exceptions to this rule might include times when the carer is too tired and distressed by the behaviour of the patient to be able to cope, or when the patient's distress is introducing a state of exhaustion detrimental to his wellbeing. A small dose of the drug chlorpromazine (Largactil) might be helpful in such circumstances.

References

Adams, K (1979) To sleep, perchance to recuperate, World Medicine, 14(22): 23

Aschoff, J (1966) Adaptive cycles, International Journal of Biometeorology, 10: 305-324

Choi-Lao, A T H (1976) The sleep assignment — a way to learn problem solving, Canadian Nurse, 72: 34-35

Clark, L (1980) Son et lumière? Nursing Mirror, 151(19): 21

Dement, W (1960) The effect of dream deprivation, Science, 131: 1705-1707

Dement, W (1974) Some Must Watch While Some Must Sleep, W H Freeman

Feinberg, I (1969) Effects of age on human sleep patterns, in A Kales (Editor) Sleep Physiology and Pathology, J B Lippincott

Garner, H G (1978) You may have to leave hospital to get well, Supervisory Nurse, 9: 76-79

Gillies, L (1976) Sleeplessness — can you help? Canadian Nurse, 72 (7): 32-34

Johnson, L C (1969) Psychological and physiological changes following total sleep deprivation, in A Kales (Editor), Sleep Physiology and Pathology, J B Lippincott

Halberg, F (1953) Some physiological and clinical aspects of twenty four hour periodicity, Lancet, 73: 20-32

Hartmann, E L (1973) The Functions of Sleep, Yale University Press

Hartmann, E L and Cravens, J (1973) The effects of long term administration of psychotropic drugs on human sleep, Psychopharmocologica, 33: 153-245

Hayter, J (1980) The rhythm of sleep, American Journal of Nursing, 80: Mar 457-461

Hilton, B A (1976) Quantity and quality of patient's sleep and sleep disturbing factors in a respiratory intensive care unit, Journal of Advanced Nursing, 1: 453-468

Hopkins, S (1980) Silent night? Nursing, 20: 870-873

Jouvet, M (1969) Biogenic amines and the states of sleep, Science, 163: 32-38

Kleitman, N (1967) Sleep and Wakefulness, University of Chicago Press

Luce, G G and Segal, J (1967) Sleep, William Heinemann

Martin, I C A (1975) Some therapeutic concepts of sleep, Nursing Times, 71(7): 1611-1614

Myco, F (1981) Circadian rhythms — clocking in? Nursing Mirror, 152(18): 32-34

Oswald, I (1980) Sleep, 4th edition, Penguin

Patrick, G (1973) Forgotten patients in medical wards, Canadian Nurse, 68(3): 27-31

Rentschaffen, A and Monroe, L J (1977) Laboratory studies of insomnia, in W B Mendleson, J C Gillin and R J Wyatt (Editors) Human Sleep and Its Disorders, Plenum Press

Schultz, L C M (1973) Nursing care of the stroke patient, Nursing Clinics of North America, 8(4): 633-641

Singer, J L (1974) Daydreaming and the stream of thought, American Scientist, 62: 417-425

Tyrer, P (1978) How to Sleep Better, Sheldon Press

Webb, W (1968) Individual differences in sleep length, International Psychiatry Clinics, 7: 44-47

Whitfield, S (1975) Noise on the ward at night, Nursing Times, 71(11): 408-412

Zelechowski, G P (1977) Helping your patients sleep — planning instead of pills, Nursing '77', 7: 62-68

CHAPTER 8

NURSING MANAGEMENT OF COMMUNICATION

Introduction

'Wa wo, you know, gonna wo — hell! shoo wo.'

These words are meaningless. They were used by a professional man, a stroke victim in his mid-fifties, to ask a passing nurse to get him a paper tissue from a box on his bedside locker. He obtained his tissue, not because the nurse understood his gibberish, but through his gesticulating towards the visible tissues. However, had he been sitting in a dayroom on the ward, or had the tissues been out of sight, his request could have been more difficult for the nurse to fulfil.

This chapter attempts to explain what communication is, why it might become disrupted in stroke, and how the nurse can help the patient, with the assistance of the speech therapist and family members.

Patrick (1973) found that nurses caring for stroke victims with speech disturbances did not appear to understand the importance of communication in their care programmes. Gough and Powell (1978b) describe a small study in which 15 patients were indicated as having 'communication difficulties', by ward sisters. Following formal testing, these stroke victims were found to have degrees of difficulty which varied with the nurse's assessment in 8 of the 15 cases. Observations showed that there was less non-verbal contact between the nurses and these patients than might have been expected. The nurses made fewer explanatory gestures, and had less eye contact with the stroke patients, compared with others in the wards. There was also a tendency among the nursing staff to move these patients around the ward or hospital without attempting any preliminary explanation. Thus, difficulties in communication among patients appear to reduce attempts at communication by nurses. Gough and Powell also claim that the nurses in this study commonly overestimated the degree of verbal understanding which the patient had. Only when they conducted simple tests did the nurses realize how little the patient understood, of what was being said. Two reasons were suggested as to why this might be. First, patients with comprehension difficulty often react appropriately to questions or instructions in the ward because of the many non-verbal cues available, e.g. knowledge of ward routine. A patient may not understand the instruction, 'open your mouth!', but he may do so spontaneously if he sees a nurse approaching him shaking a thermometer. The second suggestion arises from the lack of knowledge on the part of most nurses about the different forms of speech disorder. Most of the nursing staff, in their study, associated aphasia with some expressive difficulty, but not usually with disruption of other language modalities. When specifically asked by Gough and Powell, most of these nurses claimed that they had not been taught about the language problems of stroke patients during their training.

There is no evidence to suggest that an increase in the numbers of nursing staff will mean that more time is spent communicating with patients. Savage and Widdowson (1971) found that when more staff are available, nurses continue to give the same type of care, usually physical care, only more of it.

Regarding medical staff, Godfrey and Douglas (1959) claim that there has been an attitude of relative indifference on the part of the medical community towards recovery in aphasia, perhaps related to the notion that questions concerning recovery and rehabilitation have already been answered. Such apparent lack of interest by doctors in the performance of the aphasic patient is also mentioned by Sarno (1976). Christie and Lawrence (1978) found that while the technical skills of doctors were highly regarded by most stroke patients, their ability to communicate and relate to the stroke victim was often thought to be inadequate, especially by non-English-speaking patients. Such lack of understanding by both medical and nursing staff can have devastating consequences for the patient.

Critchley (1970) gives a striking characterization of the stroke patient who has difficulty in communication. He claims that the patient is silent most of the time.

He displays a poverty of speech. Rarely does he talk unless circumstances compel him to break silence, or try and reply to a direct question. He does not engage in conversational small talk. This is particularly noticeable when he finds himself in the company of several people. The ensuing table talk presents particular difficulties and rarely does he interpolate or contribute to the general stream of conversation. The communication net is all around him, but he remains apart. He sits quietly in his chair looking dully upon the surrounding scene; as if in a brown study. Sometimes he seems to be reading. A book or newspaper is open before him. But, as Trousseau noted some years ago, the pages are not turned; indeed sometimes the book is held upside down. The patient is not really attending to the subject matter; at the very most he is gazing vaguely at the illustrations though without full comprehension. Much of his waking time is devoted to radio and television. These pursuits constitute a pleasurable type of recreation, but rarely if ever does the patient fully comprehend the content of what he sees and hears. In all probability he does not realise his shortcomings in this respect. Testing with story telling pictures shows striking anomalies. Firstly, that the average stroke patient understands only a fraction of what is behind the pictorial theme, and secondly, the patient is unaware that something is eluding him, and that his interpretation is inadequate.

In general conversation, it is not normally necessary to ponder the next word which will be spoken. Although one might not grasp the meaning of a phrase or sentence, it is unusual to be confused by individual words within an average range of vocabulary. Finding the right word, however, can be very difficult for a stroke victim. One stroke patient explained the situation like this: 'I knew deep down what I wanted to say, but it wouldn't come out of my mouth. I felt panicky, because I couldn't make anyone understand what I wanted. They just smiled and walked away.' Accounts of personal struggles with aphasia include Moss (1972), Cameron (1973), Wulf (1973) and Dahlberg and Jaffee (1977).

To be able to offer care, a nurse must first be able to communicate with a patient. Her objective for the stroke patient should be to provide a congenial atmosphere for sensory input at a suitable level of incongruity, thereby preventing intellectual regression in the patient. Sensory input at a realistic level is essential, because as Hebb (1961) points out, repeated stimulation of specific receptors will lead slowly to the formation of an assembly of associated cells. Hebb writes: 'Any two cells or system of cells that are repeatedly active at the same time will tend to become associated so that activity in one facilitates activity in the other.' It follows that in the training of skilled responses such as writing, concern is directed to the structuring of visual, proprioceptive and auditory stimuli, with which the patient is confronted, thereby controlling the sensory input to facilitate its perception.

Disruption through a speech difficulty can be so pronounced that it can alter a patient's whole personality and, therefore, his approach to recovery. It becomes essential that the nurse's approach to communication with a stroke patient emanates from a sound knowledge base, and takes place in a therapeutic environment, which evokes a sense of team spirit. Too much stimulation and too much disorder can inhibit progress and defeat recovery.

Some aspects of communication

To say that a person has language is to imply the acquired use of symbols for the purpose of communication. Communication involves both sensory and motor elements in the understanding and use of symbols for the expression of ideas. Speech, reading and writing are learned activities, and such verbal symbols constitute the major components of communication (Figure 8.1). However, it is possible to communicate in a limited form without using words, where signs, gestures or primitive inarticulate sounds can convey information about feelings and desires.

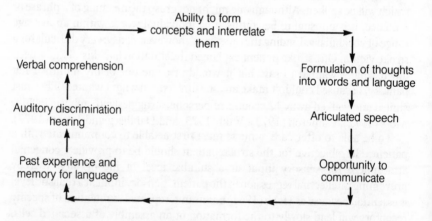

Figure 8.1 Factors in communication

The complexity of communication can lead to difficulty in defining the variegate patterns of language disorders. If the disability is severe, a disorder might be easily recognized, but subtle degrees of disorder often go undetected, even though they may be exercising a serious degree of handicap in the progress of the patient, e.g. an inability to understand the difference between 'my' and 'your', or the mixing up of the tenses, so that the future is represented in the past tense (Adams 1974). Once even a simple error makes an appearance it is extremely difficult to get rid of it, and even greater confusion can result as the patient struggles to do so.

Communication is usually classified as verbal or non-verbal. (A model of the total communication process and the central nervous system can be seen in Figure 8.2.)

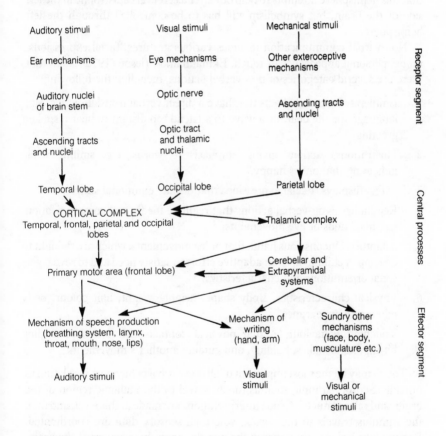

Figure 8.2 A model of communication processes and the CNS.

Verbal communication relates to the use of sound, either as words or noises. It seems likely that in 90% of people, the left hemisphere of the brain is dominant for acquiring the use of the word as a symbol. This will mean that even some left-handed people must have a dominant left hemisphere (Adams 1974), and Zangwill (1964) suggests that right hemisphere dominance may be more common in right-handed people than is usually supposed. Despite the dominance of the left hemisphere, the right side of the brain has a lead in other functions which do not involve words, such as calculation or music. It is possible that this hemisphere attempts to help out after a cerebral catastrophe in the left side of the brain, but symbolism still has to be controlled through the left hemisphere.

Non-verbal communication includes various gestures, facial expressions, mime, personal appearance or touch. Ekmann and Frieson (1975) claim that there are several categories of non-verbal actions, including the following:

1   Emblems. Non-verbal acts that have a direct verbal translation, e.g. sign language for the deaf, or a wave to a friend too distant to hear a spoken greeting.

2   Illustrations. Actions giving emphasis to words, e.g. smiling while indicating that one is happy.

3   Affect displays. Facial expressions that display emotional state.

4   Regulators. Non-verbal actions that regulate the flow of communication, e.g. head nods or eye movements.

5   Adaptors. Unconscious hand, foot or leg movements, which are thought to develop in childhood as an adaptive effort to satisfy need and to reveal personal orientations and characteristics.

6   Physical characteristics. Body shape, height, weight, hair colour, body odour and appearance.

7   Touching behaviour. Actual physical contact with others, including hitting, handshakes, holding, and guiding another's movements.

Touch may be the most important of all non-verbal behaviours in relation to nursing. Sensory stimuli, such as touch, travel to the thalamic region of the brain, and related nuclei. Crude interpretations are made at this level, and then the stimulus travels to the cortex, where all sensory data are coordinated. Parietal lobe lesions, even ones in the non-dominant hemisphere of the brain, will affect such sensory interpretations and interfere with the response of the patient to non-verbal cues (Knapp 1959). One non-verbal cue, facial expression, is difficult to evaluate without any contextual input, although there are some basic human expressions which have universal interpretation, such as smiling.

Whichever channel of communication is adopted, the individual wishing to transmit a message must first be able to encode it. The opening 'sentence' of this chapter is an example of a patient failing to do just that. The message must then be transmitted to the receiver. However, for a stimulus to effect a response, it must first be perceived (Salley and Murphey 1960). Perception follows the decoding and understanding of the message, which necessitates some function in the visual and/or auditory mechanisms, combined with cortical function along established nerve pathways in the brain. Disruption at any stage of the encoding — transmission, receiving — decoding process will result inevitably in a breakdown in communication.

If speech is to be used for communication, the transmitter must have control over his oro-laryngeal musculature, to form and project words which the receiver can decode. Also important to speech, however, is paralanguage, which deals with how something is said, rather than what is said. Elements of paralanguage include voice quality, pitch, tone, tempo and vocal characteristics such as whining, coughing or clearing the throat.

Another consideration in the process of communication is the time factor, because all behaviours take place within the dimension of time. The commitment of time can become in itself a form of communication, especially in a busy hospital department or ward. Nurses who spend unsolicited time with patients demonstrate, non-verbally, their commitment to the patient. Silence and listening are also factors to be considered. As there are positive and negative verbal transmissions, so there is positive and negative silence. Silence used constructively can help a nurse weave stronger ties with the patient (Blondis and Jackson 1977). While silence is usually passive, listening is an active process requiring understanding, skill, patience, perseverance and concentration. Perrine (1971), himself a stroke victim, claims that the nurses who cared for him could have been more helpful, by listening and giving him more time to cope in his new situation.

In conclusion, there are five general factors which might be said to contribute to an effective framework for communication. These factors can be applied to verbal communication, as follows:

1 Clarity. Avoid unfamiliar words or jargon which might confuse the receiver.

2   Brevity. Use only one idea in each sentence for transmission.

3   Simplicity. Every word should count.

4   Precision. Words which have a standard or universal meaning should be used whenever possible.

5   Integrity. The communication should avoid demanding of the receiver that he read between the lines.

Language disturbance in stroke

A stroke victim can develop difficulty with encoding messages, decoding messages or both, depending on the severity and location of the lesion in his brain. The most frightening disturbance which a stroke patient may have to endure is a sudden loss of speech or comprehension, usually known as aphasia.

Approximately 25-30% of stroke victims, notably those with right hemiplegia, suffer from aphasia (WHO 1971b). However, Nichol (1971) puts the number of patients with speech defects as high as 50%, and of these 15% would be likely to suffer both encoding and decoding disturbances, i.e. global, or total, aphasia. Gough and Powell (1978a) claim that there are at least 29 000 aphasic stroke victims in the United Kingdom at any given time, and that each year another 5200 new victims are alive 6 months after the onset of stroke. Brust et al. (1976) estimated that there are 84 000 aphasic stroke victims in the USA each year, i.e. 21% of the annual stroke occurrence.

Fortunately, 50-70% of these patients will recover some speech spontaneously. In a small study by Hagen (1973), it was found that most patients made some recovery within the first 3 months of their stroke, whether or not they received speech therapy, but after that time only those receiving therapy continued to improve.

What the nurse does about stroke in general, and aphasia in particular, will depend on what she knows about it. A historical overview may help to explain how present day theories and terminology associated with aphasia came into being.

Historical aspects of speech disorder

Aphasia was first described by the Eygptian physician Imhotep, about 3000 years BC (Sies 1974). However, the first physician to note a loss of speech in connection with stroke is said to have been Paul of Aegina (Licht 1975). Archivists have discovered that a very substantial body of knowledge about aphasia existed before the mid-nineteenth century, usually in the form of clinical descriptions (Riese 1974, Benton and Joynt 1960 and Benton 1964).

It is now universally accepted that the modern history of aphasia began with the work of the Frenchman, Paul Broca. There has been considerable argument among historians, between the supporters of Broca and those of Marc Dax, over the question of priority. Dax, also a Frenchman, claimed that he associated loss of speech with right hemiplegia 25 years before Broca, in 1836. However, it appears that the work of Dax, like that of other forerunners, was at best an isolated flash of insight, which set no new activities in motion (Geschwind 1974).

The 'localization' argument

Broca's work had its origins in evidence of the effect of electrical stimulation on the cerebral cortex, ideas which were first advanced by Franz Gall in 1813. Paul Broca presented his renowned paper to the Académie de la Société d'Anthropologie in Paris in 1861. This paper, 'Remarques sur le siège de la faculté du langage articulé suivies d'une observation d'aphémie (perte de la parole)', is important because it was the first formal mention of the relation between brain disorder and language loss. Included in this description (Broca 1861a) of two cases of patients with cerebral injury was this paragraph:

Aphemia, that is to say, loss of speech, results from a lesion of the frontal lobe of the brain . . . the primary site of the lesions was in the second or third convolution; most probably in the latter in all cases . . . [This] puts aside for the present the idea that the linguistic faculty resides in a fixed point.

The word aphemia was replaced by aphasia when it was pointed out that in ancient times aphemia meant infantile.

It has been claimed, however, that both of Broca's patients were of advanced age, and damage to the left hemisphere, from other causes, was extensive in both cases (Osgood and Miron 1970). Nevertheless, later in 1861, Broca claimed that the third convolution of the left frontal lobe was indispensable to articulated speech (Broca 1861b). These articles, fixing specific centres in the brain as being the seat of language, stimulated and directed the thinking and research of most neurologists for decades afterwards (Wepman 1951). Broca's research into the structure of the third convolution of the left hemisphere led to the adoption of the name 'Broca's area' for that part of the brain. The expressive language defect which he described became known as 'Broca's aphasia'.

Broca's work was immediately taken up in England, by Bastian, who was among the first to use diagrams to illustrate localization theories. Through his intricate diagrams, Bastian claimed to be able to show the exact location of a particular lesion which was producing the language behaviour which was being observed (Bastian 1880). He divided all language problems into two groups: those involving difficulties of comprehension; and those involving difficulty with speaking.

In 1864, a 26 year old German neurologist, Carl Wernicke, published his first study of the brain. He described an auditory centre in the first temporal convolution as being the receiving, or 'sensory', zone of the brain (Wernicke 1874). He agreed with Broca that the frontal convolution was the centre for articulated language, but maintained that the temporal convolution was the location for the reception of auditory impulses on the level of comprehension. Wernicke's work was so widely accepted that this temporal convolution in the left hemisphere was called 'Wernicke's area', and the type of language defect involved 'Wernicke's aphasia'.

Other neurologists began to claim discovery of language centres all over the brain. Another early pioneer of localization theory, J M Charcot, developed the idea of a writing or graphic centre in the brain. He also believed there was a centre for 'ideation', which served as an integrating force for all other 'centred' cortical activity. While such theories are no longer universally accepted, Charcot was among the first to observe the differences in behaviour of patients suffering from the same or similar neurological defects. From such observations, he postulated there would be different kinds of individuals, e.g. some would be 'auditory minded' and others 'visually minded' (Charcot and Pitres 1883). In 1895, Charcot labelled the middle cerebral artery, the 'apoplexy artery', because of its frequent involvement in stroke (Licht 1975).

Localization theory reached its peak at the turn of the century, through the papers of Charles Mills. He attempted to differentiate precise structural zones for a motor centre, an auditory-speech centre, a visual centre and a graphic or writing centre (Mills 1904). He mistakenly attempted to attribute the intellectual component in aphasia to sensorial causes. However, he was among the first to view the practical aspects of aphasia, its medical considerations and the concept of treatment by speech therapy. The first reference to re-education of aphasics is attributed to Hunt (1851) and supported by Baleman (1890).

The theories of localization began to wane as the science of psychology emerged. Nevertheless, a formal structural approach to mental activity still finds some support among neurologists today. Figure 8.3 shows some of the areas of the brain which have been linked with language function.

Figure 8.3 The language areas of brain

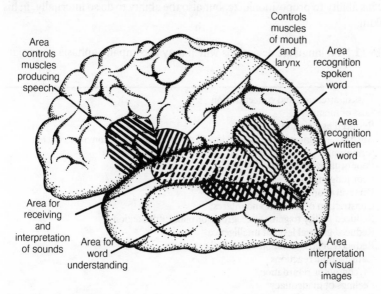

Controls muscles of mouth and larynx

Area controls muscles producing speech

Area recognition spoken word

Area recognition written word

Area for receiving and interpretation of sounds

Area for word understanding

Area interpretation of visual images

The non-localization argument

The 'diagram makers', as localizationists were often nicknamed, were criticized on the grounds of inadequate data and inadequate theory. In 1906, Pierre Marie re-examined the preserved brains of Broca's patients, and demonstrated the fallacy of attributing single symptoms to circumscribed lesions in such generally deteriorated brains (Marie 1906). He described the non-language behaviour of the brain-injured adult, e.g. problems of inattention and amnesia or memory loss. (A more comprehensive list of non-verbal behaviour associated with aphasia is offered in Table 11.)

Interest in the work of Marie led to the rediscovery of the writings of the Englishman, John Hughlings Jackson. Working at the same time as Broca, Jackson formulated a concept of the dynamic behaviour of the individual. He believed that the defect involved in post-traumatic language problems concerned the individual's ability to 'propositionalize'. This means the ability to draw and redraw relationships between individual words which will give them a new meaning. He claimed that single words are meaningless, and that the unit of speech is not the word, but the proposition formed by the interaction of all words used (Jackson 1931). He believed that in aphasia the patient loses not only his ability to propositionalize, but also the ability to do so internally, in his thinking.

Table 11 Non language deviations which may accompany aphasia (Wepman 1951)

1	Loss of attention and concentration
2	Loss of memory
3	Reduced association of ideas
4	Abstract — concrete imbalance (loss of ability to abstract, concrete concept formation)
5	Poor organizing ability
6	Poor judgement
7	Perseveration
8	Constriction of thought and interest
9	Reduced ability to generalize, group or plan future action
10	Reduced general level of intelligence
11	Reduced ability to inhibit emotional responses
12	Catastrophic reactions
13	Psychomotor retardation
14	Feelings of inadequacy
15	Egocentricity; disinterest in both human and physical environment
16	Fatigue and irritability
17	Euphoria
18	Social withdrawal and seclusiveness
19	Reduced ability to adjust to new situations
20	Reduced initiative and spontaneity
21	Externalization of behaviour; a lack of self-criticism
22	Automatic verbalization
23	Impulsive, regressive behaviour
24	Anxiety and tension
25	Changing personality profile
26	Hemiplegia

Lecturing just 3 years after Broca's famous paper, Jackson warned that speech and words are psychical terms. While words must have an anatomical basis, the memory of words cannot be localized to any part of the nervous system. He was the first to realize the importance of a psychological approach to the understanding of the problems of an aphasic patient, long before psychological theory as we know it today began to evolve. Hughlings Jackson's second important contribution was that he introduced the idea that the dissolution of the nervous system, after stroke, shows a hierarchy of breakdown of functional levels. The higher levels, which evolve later in our development, break down first in the dissolution process. He also described aphasic patients using 'automatic' speech, although still incapable of expressing a proposition.

The theory that language dissolution presents as a reversal of the pattern of normal language development has been pursued by Wepman (1951), and Jakobson and Halle (1956). They suggest that the most complex forms of language, which develop last, are usually the first to be lost in aphasia (Table 12). Consequently, the more primitive the language form which the patient uses, the more critical will have been the damage inflicted on the speech areas of the brain.

Table 12 Dissolution of language in aphasia (after Jakobson and Halle 1956)

Direction of normal language development	Stage	Type of speech	Stage of language development
	1	Global	Pre-language: characterized by speechlessness
	2	Jargon	Pre-language: characterized by meaningless, autistic and echoic phenomena
	3	Pragmatic	Progressive acquistion of comprehension; oral expression of words and neologisms largely unrelated to meaning or below level of comprehension
	4	Semantic	Beginning use of substantive language, progressing through nominal, verbal and adjectival words; characterized by one or two word groups as a complete expression
	5	Syntactic	Use of syntax or grammar in oral expression
			Direction of language dissolution in aphasia

The importance of considering total cortical activity for language and thought was sustained by Jackson's students in England (e.g. Gowers 1885). Pierre Marie continued to support Jacksonian theory in France. In 1922, he was the first to recognize that aphasia was not limited in its language deficit to the area of speech, but that such a deficit extended to every part of the communication act, including pantomime (Marie 1922). Total cortical integration theory gained momentum through the support of neurologist Arnold Pick, in Czechoslovakia, and psychologist Sigmund Freud in Austria. However, it was the work of Henry Head in England that gave direction and analysis to the work of Jackson, which forms the basis of present day thinking (Wepman 1951). Head emphasized the problems of abstract thinking which aphasics suffer. He devised a series of language tests which he administered to patients with a diversity of symptoms (Head 1926).

The development of Gestalt psychology, through the work of Kohler and others, contributed to something of an over-reaction to localization theory in the 1930s. Collecting material for studies in perception, psychologists postulated that cerebral regions, areas or fields, and not specific sites, are responsible for the function of the brain. The supporters of such propositions became known as field theorists, and their ideas received the support of such prominent neurologists as Kurt Goldstein (1939).

Several other studies promote the theory of non-localization. For example, Conrad (1954) observed 216 aphasic patients, and demonstrated that the lesions in their brains, even if eventually localized, were still widely scattered over the dominant hemisphere and produced different types of aphasia. Penfield and Roberts (1959), through the use of electrical stimulation to conscious human brains, claimed that the results which they obtained demonstrated the presence of at least one supplementary expressive area in the cortex. Consequently, if one of the main speech areas is destroyed, adjacent areas take over. Finally, Weisenberg and McBride (1964) claimed that the locality of the lesion in the aphasic patients whom they studied could not account for the clinical manifestations of language dysfunction which they observed. Recent developments in technology, such as brain scanning, are providing evidence which supports the inspired insights of Jackson, but the issue is by no means finally resolved.

The Jacksonian principles which dictate modern approaches to aphasia have been summed up by Wepman (1951) in the following way:

1   There is no commonly defined area in the cortex for the centre for language.

2   Observation of the patient takes precedence over anatomical data.

3   The concepts of higher and lower language behaviour should be applied to individuals with aphasia.

4   The theory of dissolution can be applied to the behaviour in these patients.

5   It has to be recognized that non-language factors are also disturbed in aphasia.

6   There should be an appreciation of the close relationship between thought and language, but with an understanding that they are not one and the same thing.

In summary, it has been established that there is 'localization' of language functions, in the gross sense that one hemisphere, usually the left, is dominant. Whether this means that speech functions in the normal individual are entirely organized in the left hemisphere, or simply that the left side is dominant in control over the final expressive pathways, is by no means certain (Osgood and Miron 1970). The evidence of spontaneous recovery indicates that there must be some replication of function, either between the two hemispheres, or between regions of the dominant hemisphere. The reason why localization and non-localization arguments are important rests in the direction which they give to the recovery process to be adopted. A more hopeful prognosis can be made for aphasic stroke victims through the acceptance of the non-localization viewpoint, according to which recovery follows reintegration of the remaining cortical tissue into a functioning whole.

Classification of aphasia

Early attempts at providing definitions for the symptoms of language disturbance tended to be very broad and not very helpful. For example, Kussmaul (1877) claimed aphasia was, 'the impairment of execution, expression, or understanding of any symbols by which man communicates his ideas or feelings to others'. More recently, Taylor (1964a) used the term aphasia to mean, 'an acquired impairment of verbal behaviour caused by brain damage, which impedes the linguistic features in encoding or decoding language'. DeVito (1970) also stresses a disruption in the manipulation of the encoding and decoding abilities of the patient. Similarly, Osgood and Miron (1970) define aphasia as, 'a non functional impairment in the reception, manipulation and/or expression of symbolic content whose basis is to be found in organic damage to relatively central brain structure'.

However, one of the most dynamic and functional definitions of aphasia has been put forward by Schuell et al. (1964), who claim that, 'aphasia is a language deficit that crosses all language modalities, characterised by impaired verbal retention span, the reduction of functional vocabulary, and the impairment of perception, and the production of messages'.

Aphasia, or absence of language, is not a strictly precise term, because at least one utterance is usually present, if only part of a word or intelligible noise. Dysphasia, or difficulty with language, is a more exact term. However, in present-day literature, aphasia and dysphasia are used synonymously. Aphasia will be used throughout this text.

Whatever the preferred definition, the term aphasia can be confusing because it is used to refer to infinite numbers and types of impairment. Its use should exclude all those communication disorders due to neuromuscular impairment, dysfunction of the peripheral sense organs, mental deficiency, organic mental syndromes and psychpathology. While deficiencies in writing, gesture, calculation and reading frequently accompany aphasia, isolated losses in such skills, without concurrent encoding/decoding dysfunction, do not independently constitute an aphasic syndrome.

The term aphasia is problematic in that, when used by itself, it does not indicate the degree of impairment, the linguistic features which are impaired, a prognosis for recovery or a method of treatment (Taylor 1964b).

Many attempts have been made to classify aphasia, and the value of such classifications is frequently challenged. For example, Buck (1970), himself a stroke victim, claims that from his own experience there is no possible means for measuring how accurately or how well the patient can understand the words he hears. He explains that, following his stroke, he had moments or hours of good perception, mixed with days of lack of understanding.

Despite their shortcomings, the classifications of aphasia in the literature tend to adopt one of two forms. First, the classical categorization system of expressive, receptive and global aphasia, and second, the system using the terms fluent, non-fluent and global aphasia, as expounded by Geschwind (1970b), Kerschensteiner et al. (1972) and Wagenaar et al. (1975). These are simply two different terminologies for the same phenomena, in that the words expressive and receptive are more or less synonymous with non-fluent and fluent. Brust et al. (1976) point out, however, that it is not always easy to classify speech as fluent or non-fluent. Because of the complexity of the various terminologies adopted by different authors, the classical system will be used in this text.

The words expressive or receptive are used to qualify when the patient's aphasia tends to cluster in encoding (expressive) or decoding (receptive) language skills, or both (global).

Expressive aphasia (also known as motor, non-fluent or Broca's aphasia)
The stroke victim with expressive aphasia has difficulty making himself understood, in both speech and writing. However, he will have retained a good comprehension for words, so he will be able to understand what is being said to him, and he will be able to read messages. Why this occurs is by no means fully understood. Gazzaniga and Sperry (1967) claim that the right hemisphere of the brain can comprehend symbols even when the patient is unable to name them, because the lesion is cutting off the right hemisphere from the word store in the left hemisphere. Thus, if a symbol such as a clenched fist is flashed into the left half of the patient's vision, so that it travels only to the right hemisphere of the brain, he may be able to perform the gesture adequately, but not be able to put into words what the picture suggested he should do. The work of Geschwind (1965 and 1970a) demonstrates there are several expressive aphasic syndromes. For example, syndromes which arise from lesions affecting the cortical connections within the hemispheres, or across the corpus callosum connecting the two sides of the brain. He calls the patients suffering from these disorders, 'disconnexion aphasics', and while they have good comprehension and their ability to speak remains good, they are unable to repeat words spoken by others.

Occasionally patients with severe encoding problems have some *automatic* speech, such as counting or recalling the days of the week or nursery rhymes, but they are not able to use these words functionally. Another form of automatic speech is swearing. Profanity can be included in the patient's verbalizations regardless of his previous history of swearing, and it can be uttered with a cordial tone of voice, a sad one, or in a tone of irritability, often out of character for the patient. Such utterances may last for months, sometimes in combination with the expression of meaningful phrases. Gradually the swearing may disappear, except in periods of extreme fatigue (Buck 1970). If the patient or his family show distress at his profanities, it should be explained that this is one of the symptoms of his aphasia, which will usually subside as the patient achieves a broader vocabulary of words.

Relatives may also be puzzled as to why a patient who cannot speak can sing old songs with apparent ease. He can do this because the centre for music and singing lies in the unaffected right hemisphere. To demonstrate this phenomenon, try this simple exercise. Recall the third line of the national anthem — now! For most people the recall of the words of the third line will only be possible by recalling the tune to which they are 'attached', that is, singing the anthem to oneself to get to the required words. There is no need for abstract thought to retrieve this information.

The expressive aphasic tends to be very reluctant in his speech. Because his comprehension of language is relatively unimpaired, he will be aware that he is making mistakes, and this will inhibit his attempts to speak. The patient will tend to use nouns by themselves, without other parts of speech, e.g. 'bed' instead of 'going to bed', or he may only use 'yes' or 'no' on every possible occasion (Gough and Powell 1978a). He frequently mispronounces words, and has difficulty putting any connected utterances together (Geschwind 1970b). Language impairment following stroke worsens with advancing age, and the elderly do not respond so well to therapy as other age groups (Mitchell 1958, Vignolo 1964, Smith 1971, and Kersetz and McCabe 1977).

Anomia, also known as amnesic or nominal aphasia, is a term used in relation to word-finding difficulty. At times we all experience the frustration of being unable to find the right word, but this is a persistent problem for the aphasic patient. It is an impairment which may persist as a residual problem long after spontaneous recovery has been achieved in other aspects of speech (Quinting 1971).

The hesitant speech of a typical expressive aphasia patient is both slurred and strikingly deficient in all words, especially prepositions. Grammar is deranged and sticking on a particular word is common. The same mistakes tend to be made if naming is nearly correct (Adams 1974). Perseveration is also common, but may be limited to parts of words, e.g. cigarrrette. Sometimes two words may be combined into a new word or neologism, for example, pipe and cigarette = cigapipe.

When the main feature of disordered speech is naming difficulty, *periphrasis* might also occur. This is when the patient circumvents the difficulty by describing the use of the object, rather than naming it. For example, 'glass' for 'drink', or 'pen' for 'write'. Another example of periphrasis is when the patient chooses the wrong word, but one which is in a related class, e.g., 'sheet' for 'bed'. Alternatively, his efforts may result in a new word possessing some connection in sound or meaning, e.g. bath becomes 'a path dipper'.

Expressive aphasia should not be confused with *dysarthria*. This is a collective term for a group of speech disorders resulting from disturbances in muscular control over the speech mechanism. The patient's problem in oral communication is due to paralysis, weakness or incoordination in the speech musculature (Schow et al. 1978). It occurs in stroke involving the basilar artery, which results in damage to the brain stem. Consequently, the speech of the patient can become very slurred. Flaccidity in the muscles of the throat and mouth leads to a hypernasal resonant quality of the voice, with a nasal emission. Weakness of the lips and tongue develops imprecise consonants, a reduced articulatory rate and unintelligibility.

Receptive aphasia (also known as sensory, fluent or Wernicke's aphasia)

While even a severe expressive aphasic patient can regain social independence, this is not easy to achieve for the patient who has difficulty in comprehension or decoding (Adams and Hurwitz 1963, Kenin and Swisher 1972).

Receptive aphasia, which is usually associated with posterior cerebral lesions, may be severe or selective. There might be a combination of factors, including no comprehension of words and an inability to repeat words and to read or write; neither can such a patient tell the time. Occasionally, there are outpourings of nonsense language, known as jargon aphasia (Adams 1974). The patient is rarely aware of the nonsense that he is talking. To empathize with the situation of the patient, try to imagine what it must feel like to wake up suddenly and find yourself surrounded by people speaking a language you don't understand.

The patient is relatively eager to talk, and his speech will be normal in rhythm and tone, although there is some tendency to speak rapidly. There should be no hesitancy as in expressive aphasia, but he often rambles and uses jargon, because he doesn't understand what he is saying. Consequently, he cannot maintain his own speech performance for long. He has no difficulty using verbs, adverbs and adjectives, as well as nouns. In addition, he may be able to name objects, but will tend to describe them in terms of their use. Although his speech performance may be basically capable, semantic and syntactic elements may be disrupted. Receptive aphasia is commonly associated with homonymous hemianopia and proprioceptive loss on the right side.

Global aphasia (also known as total aphasia)

The patient with global aphasia will have impairment of all aspects of language function and, therefore, will have lost practically all opportunity to communicate; a truly catastrophic situation for him. He may be left with only a single word or utterance, and he cannot understand gestures, or comprehend the spoken word, or read or write. In global aphasia, the expressive defect rarely improves, but some degree of comprehension may become re-established in time. His speech, if it does improve, is unlikely to progress beyond jargon. While the nurse should not present a pessimistic outlook, she should caution the relatives not to become over-optimistic when the patient shows early signs of improvement. The first sign of recovery tends to be in the use of echoic responses. These are primitive verbalizations, which are not strongly structured because of poor perception. This type of distorted self-talk, often mistaken for dementia, may be the patient's way of fixing percepts from one experience to the next (Buck 1970).

The prognosis is poor, and speech therapy is not normally indicated for this type of aphasia.

Reading and writing

The brain-damaged adult cannot consistently perceive the whole of anything (Buck 1970). He finds it difficult to distinguish figure from background, substance from shadow, or patterns, to the extent that comprehension becomes distorted. The result can be an endless sequence of misconception, so the patient needs time to re-establish some order for the promotion of his understanding.

An expressive aphasic will lose his ability to write and spell, a receptive aphasic loses his ability to read and understand, while a global aphasic will lose all abilities in written communication. In this situation, it is extremely important to wait until the patient with expressive aphasia indicates a wish to read a magazine or newspaper. After all, many adults do not read recreationally. Nearly 2 000 000 adults in Britain have a reading age of nine, or under, and would not want their semi-illiteracy exposed. To push a patient too quickly into attempting to read, especially if contrary to his normal habit, could demoralize him. If the patient with expressive aphasia is unable to organize oral communication, it seems ridiculous to have him make attempts to express himself by the written word. Unfortunately, it is not uncommon to see a well-intentioned nurse encouraging a patient to write. The patient who cannot write is said to have agraphia. Examples of speech and writing problems associated with expressive aphasia can be seen in Table 13.

Many stroke victims, especially the elderly, may feel they have no need to write. Therefore, it would seem pointless to traumatize the right hemiplegic with the failures of left-handed script. Writing should not be enforced as an alternative method of communication in aphasia, rather the nurse should wait until the patient indicates a willingness to try. As a rule, writing should be the very last procedure to be introduced.

Table 13 Problems of speech and writing in expressive aphasia

1	Cannot remember how to spell a word
2	Substitutes or omits letters of words, e.g. Danube = Dnbe bank = brank
3	Transposes letters of words, e.g. train = trian dust = dsut
4	Substitues associated words, e.g. cup = teapot sock = shoe
5	Substitutes similar words, e.g. coat = boat lift = shift
6	Persists with a previously written word (perseveration), even if he knows that it is wrong
7	Perseveration of a previously written letter, e.g. petrol = petrool bread = brrread
8	To aid recollection, traces letters with finger
9	If bilingual, may substitue word of the more recently learned language e.g. house = maison pound = punt
10	Tries to recognize a word by speaking individual letters at beginning of word, and then guesses remainder, e.g. below = be-long whistle = wh-isker
11	Tries to identify words through phonetics to aid defective visual recall, so words with silent or double letters are frequently mis-spelled

Prognosis

Schuell et al. (1964) devised the Minnesota Test for Differential Diagnosis of Aphasia, which they claim provides more objective diagnostic and prognostic information than any other method of aphasic examination. They devised the classification system for prognosis illustrated in Table 14.

Nursing assessment of aphasia

While an understanding of some of the physical, pathological and clinical aspects of aphasia is essential, the nurse is ultimately concerned with the effect which the condition has on a patient's ability to communicate. Communication, therefore, has to be understood, not in isolation, but in the context which encompasses the total personality and external reality of the patient (Schwab

Table 14 Comparison of the characteristics and prognosis of aphasic groups and syndromes (Schuell et al. 1964)

Group	Designation	Prognosis
1*	Simple aphasia; reduction of language in all modalities in the absence of any specific motor or sensori-motor involvement	Excellent
2*	Aphasia with cerebral involvement of the visual processes (e.g. hemianopia)	Excellent for language not dependent on visual processes; recovery is slowest in reading and writing
3	Aphasia with sensori-motor involvement (e.g. hemiplegia)	Limited, but functional recovery of language possible
4	Aphasia with visual and motor involvement	Speech therapy is still indicated
5	Irreversible aphasia syndrome with almost complete loss of functional language skills in all modalities (e.g. global)	Poor prognosis; since any gains do not become functional, e.g. patient remains unable to ask for a glass of water when he wants it. Only limited and realistic short-term speech therapy is indicated

* Unlikely to be admitted to hospital.

1972). While the degree of disability in aphasia follows a very broad spectrum, only the more severely involved patients will present nursing management problems (Hirschberg et al. 1976). Nevertheless, an assessment should be carried out on all stroke patients to identify any language dysfunction, for what might not present a 'nursing' problem may still be detrimental to the patient's welfare, particularly when he leaves hospital.

The nurse's ability to conduct an assessment is one of the critical factors in the recovery of the patient. Such an assessment is not easily conducted, because it demands the willing and total co-operation of the patient. The expected rules of behaviour may be simply ignored by the patient. For example, stroke victim Buck (1970), relates that his carers assumed 'yes' meant that he understood, but he claims that, 'many times I nodded my head, *simply to get rid of them*'.

Setting up communication

Brain cells once destroyed do not regenerate, so the success or failure of attempts to restore speech may depend upon the therapeutic measures taken. Appropriate measures can be undertaken only after identification of the basic factors responsible for the various symptoms, and recognition of the means whereby the defects may be compensated for (Luria 1970).

If the power of speech is lost, or markedly impaired, and the power of writing gone, the nurse can no longer hear or see the mind of the patient at work in the way she is accustomed to do (Whittet 1971). This can be very bewildering for both the nurse and the patient. Yet it would be wrong to assume that the patient is completely unaware of his plight. He is still a person and a personality, and he will still be feeling things deeply, but without an ability to express them. This may well lead to an apparent irritability, intolerance or restlessness, or even outbursts of rage or gloomy depression in the patient, because he has suddenly been deprived of the usual safety valve which we all use to give vent to our feelings. However, it would be wrong to assume that all anxiety or sadness displayed by the patient is maladaptive and calls for nursing intervention. Professional intervention is necessary only when anxiety is significantly discomforting. Emotional response should be assessed on the basis of its degree and its reasonableness under the given circumstances (Altmann 1972).

The nurse requires information as to how the aphasic patient is coping with his situation, so it behoves her to observe his day-to-day, hour-to-hour, verbal and non-verbal activity. She should note how much of the 24 hours he sleeps, what exactly he does with his waking hours, and what he tries to say.

Communication, and the rehabilitation of its disorders, thrives on a consistent environment, and understanding, considerate people. Buck (1970) claims that there were three major environmental shortcomings in his hospital care, which the nurses might have paid attention to. In the placement of his bed, no allowance was made for his 'blind' side, so he could not see anyone to talk to. In addition, placing him among ill patients gave him no incentive to talk. The second obstacle was that after the morning care round was complete, he was usually left sitting at his bedside, facing no one. Finally, he claims that when family consultations were arranged, they tended to be 'too casual' and 'too boring' for him to feel the urge to join in.

The nurse should not only take notes on what the patient says, but what are the circumstances which prompted him to speak. Sometimes the patient may make things up, in order to please the nurse or carer. He may make misleading statements simply because he is tired, bored, inattentive or in a depressed state.

Some form of communication should be established as soon as the consciousness of the patient has cleared. All sensory modalities, including gesture and mime, should be tried in the search for the most fruitful method of communication. Bright (1972) advocates the value of music when other forms of communication are not successful. Indeed, Luria et al. (1965) cite the case of a Russian composer who wrote his best work after suffering global aphasia. A charge nurse told me about an Irish woman in long-term care, who had sat passive and mute for as long as anyone could remember. One day a nurse introduced some records of traditional Irish music, and to everyone's surprise, the woman walked to the centre of the room, danced a jig and sat down again.

The rhythm of poetry might also be explored. Critchley (1970) cites several examples of poetic creativity in aphasia.

The decision as to when and how to treat the patient's aphasia is usually made by the speech therapist, on the basis of results from special tests. However, the progress of the patient cannot rest solely on the input of the speech therapist, because he will require a lot of stimulation in communication from the beginning of his recovery period. Hirschberg et al. (1976) claim that such stimulation will reduce the shock of the patient's first confrontation with his communication problems, and help prevent him developing negative compensatory approaches, such as withdrawal and failure to try. Such bad habits, once established, take a lot of effort to undo, and may prevent the patient reaching his predicted level of recovery.

Even when speech therapy services are in short supply, every stroke patient is entitled to at least a reasonable therapeutic trial (Rosenthal 1971).

Failure and frustration in other areas of disability can complicate the assessment and rehabilitation of language dysfunction. Factors for predicting improvement in communication include perceptual loss, low motivation, confused and disorientated thinking, withdrawn apathetic behaviour, extended time since onset of stroke, previous stroke, low blood pressure and extended period of unconsciousness at the time of the stroke (Anderson et al. 1974).

Favourable linguistic factors in aphasia include the following:

1   Left handedness in the patient; because he is more likely to have language function in both hemispheres.

2   Under 60 years of age.

3   Any receptive impairment is mild, or absent.

4   Non verbal communication is adequate.

5   There is no accompanying neurological disease.

If there is hemiplegia and loss of feeling on his affected side, the patient may not be able to interpret directional instructions. For example, forwards, backwards, sideways to right or left, are terms which may not be easily understood.

Linguists have long recognized that spoken language produced in natural situations is markedly different in its linguistic characteristics from language which is elicited through questioning or testing (Taylor 1965). This phenomenon remains the same following stroke. This does not mean that natural everyday language is random, rather that it obeys its own, different set of rules. The disorders of language display their own particular order and, consequently, require a systematic linguistic comparison with normal verbal codes (DeReuck and O'Connor 1964). When a nurse, or therapist, asks the patient to try and write his name, he is performing a clinical act, since a task has been presented to him. On the other hand, when he signs a letter or a cheque, he is performing functionally, and his language behaviour is natural to the situation. Consequently, his assessment should not be composed of clinical tasks alone, but should include any aspect of the patient's activities in a normal situation.

The role of the speech therapist

The speech therapist has a vital role in establishing a non-verbal language where verbal communication remains poor (Patterson 1971). She helps the aphasic patient by being an interpreter and social link, forming a bridge between the patient and those around him, especially in the early days of his problem. This aspect of her work, linked with that of assessment of the patient's defect, is the primary function of the speech therapist in the treatment of stroke (Leche 1974). Another function of the speech therapist is to give instruction to relatives and staff concerning speech and phonation (Roaf and Hodkinson 1977).

The work of the speech therapist can be particularly effective during the period of spontaneous recovery. Butterfield and Zangwill (1946), following experimental studies, established that there is a spontaneous recovery period for aphasia, and that early therapy renders significantly greater language ability in those who receive it. Vignolo (1964) claims that most spontaneous recovery takes place in the first 2 months post stroke, and that therapy has a specific positive effect if it is continued for at least 6 months. Kersetz and McCabe (1977) write that the recovery rate in aphasia is clearly related to the time of examination or testing, and the introduction of therapy. This is supported by Basso et al. (1975). In addition, Policoff (1970) suggests that speech therapy should begin as soon as the patient is in physiological balance, and his life is no longer at risk. These and other studies verify the following:

1 The time period from injury to therapy is an important and significant factor in recovery from aphasia.

2 Speech therapy has the greatest possible effect when coincidental with spontaneous recovery.

3 Intensive therapy has a positive effect on recovery.

Early assessment and intensive therapy, the value of which is clearly demonstrated, are not always introduced in practice. Brocklehurst et al. (1978) carried out a study of 135 patients 2 weeks after their stroke. Aphasia was present in 39 patients (29%), dysarthria in 45 patients (35%), and both aphasia and dysarthria in 8 patients (6%). However, only 19 patients received speech therapy, i.e. 25% of the aphasic/dysarthric group. 9 of these patients received speech therapy for less than 9 days, and only 5 patients continued therapy for more than 30 days. Only 3 patients discontinued therapy because of good progress. Other reasons for discontinuation were: discharged or transferred (4 patients); no progress (6 patients); and died or other reason (2 patients). This study also showed that 75% of these patients did not begin therapy until more than 2 weeks after their stroke.

Garraway et al. (1980) compared the progress of stroke patients treated in medical wards with those cared for in stroke units. They claim that there was no difference in the level of recovery from aphasia following therapy among patients treated in either setting. Only 13% of the patients in the stroke unit, and 18% in the medical ward, received any speech therapy. In the stroke unit, the mean delay for starting therapy was 9 days and the mean duration of therapy was 61 days, but the mean number of therapy hours recorded was only 17 per patient. In the medical wards the means were 6 days, 65 days, and 11 hours respectively. This study shows that although speech therapy commenced fairly quickly in a small number of stroke patients, and lasted over 2 months, there was a lack of the intensity which is stated as being desirable.

Gough and Powell (1978b), from a limited study, claim that referral for speech therapy varies greatly. Even when the ward sister claimed that referral was 'routine', they found no evidence in either the case notes of the patient, or the speech therapy department, that it had actually been made. They claim, 'referral was initiated solely by the ward sister, and this reflected the doctor's view of stroke rehabilitation, and the efficiency of speech therapy'. One criticism which can be made against these studies is that they do not record the ages of the various patient groups.

The age of the patient should be taken into account as a part of the overall assessment. If the patient is over 70 years of age intensive speech therapy courses are generally inappropriate, but they would be essential for a few survivors, particularly for those still able to work (Weddell and Beresford 1979).

The absence of a speech therapist should not be an excuse for failure to work on the communication problem of the patient, since a nurse, family member or volunteer can be pressed into service, with good results, if patience and repetitious verbal exercise at simple levels are carried out for prolonged periods of care (Policoff 1970). Most of all the patient needs to gain confidence that he will be listened to, and the value of relatives and volunteers should not be underestimated in this respect (Meickle et al. 1979).

Factors in assessment

Each aphasic patient is a different person, and he may have a predominant difficulty in one aspect of language or another. Nevertheless, any assessment of a speech disturbance should take place against a background of information which includes the following:

1   Relevant medical history, e.g. any residual defect (such as hemiplegia), tests for hearing and visual acuity, and any loss of facial muscle power which might affect the fitting of dentures.
2   Emotional history, e.g. the patient's premorbid personality, any emotional lability or confusional state.
3   Social background, e.g. his relationships in the ward and at home, or his premorbid vocabulary and numeracy levels.

A premorbid assessment in language proficiency, estimated according to known social, educational and personality factors in the patient's history, represents a base against which change can be measured. Such a profile is necessary because an assessment by a speech therapist may require several visits to the patient, and his language abilities can alter as the result of changes in his physical or emotional state, the degree of fatigue, the effects of drugs, or any specific situation (Meikle 1981). A specific situation might be one where the patient cannot sit correctly and remain comfortable, with the result that he cannot concentrate on his speech for very long. The premorbid profile helps the speech therapist to make a more accurate assessment of the patient's situation.

The success of the assessment could also depend on the way the nurse or therapist approaches the patient. Aphasic patients respond better to clear, slow speech, within a well-defined context (Gardner et al. 1975). This does not mean that the speaker should use childish speech or shout. Very few patients acquire deafness after stroke. Short sentences and single commands are often easier for the patient to cope with, especially in the early stages of recovery.

The environment in which the assessment is to take place demands careful consideration. Quietness and privacy are essential. Patients cannot compete with radio, television, traffic noise, interruptions by staff and the general background distractions of a hospital ward (Rolnick and Hoops 1969). I recently witnessed a speech therapist vainly struggling for 20 minutes to gain the attention of an aphasic patient, whose bed was directly opposite the nurse's station, where all manner of distractions were taking place. This patient showed definite signs of embarrassment as the therapist pushed picture cards into his face, with other patients looking on. Such an environment was not conducive to an accurate assessment of that particular patient's language dysfunction.

While the formal assessment is usually carried out by the speech therapist, the role of the nurse and family members should be given a greater emphasis than is reflected in the literature, because the totality of the patient's situation cannot be understood by a few minutes of formal testing. As Hurwitz and Adams (1972) have pointed out, no one seems to be able, as yet, to define criteria of assessment to separate those who will benefit from speech therapy from those who will not. They claim that any language assessment should include the following:

1   Visual contact which the patient makes with people and objects.

2   Sound location, e.g. turns his head in response to sound.

3   Hand and eye coordination, e.g. his willingness to reach for objects.

4   Ability to imitate the mouthing of words.

5   Response to simple mime.

6   Response to repetitive speech to indicate:
   a.   If the soft palate is working.
   b.   The extent of possible articulation.
   c.   Whether normal voice is available.
   d.   Whether language is complicated by jargon.

7   Penmanship, and ability to sign his name.

8   Capacity to respond to pictures, and written words.

Hurwitz and Adams (1972) claim that the fact that patients with poor comprehension do badly so often may be because those responsible for them are given no opportunity to develop alternative means of communication, such as mime, which may pass for words. Society, both medical and lay, is very word-orientated. Not all aphasic patients will have an opportunity to receive speech therapy, and many who do so will not respond to it. It would appear that many of the techniques currently used for assessment and treatment in aphasia do not allow for cost-effective use of limited resources. Furthermore, current training programmes for nurses do not appear to be providing them with the necessary techniques to help aphasic patients who do not receive speech therapy, for whatever reason.

Tests for aphasia

In recent years many so-called aphasic tests have been designed and developed to discover and describe what language a patient has retained in speech, writing and similar modalities. Consequently, the speech therapist has a number of formal assessment tools to help her in her work. For example, some such as the Porch Index of Communicative Ability, concentrate on auditory discrimination, while others are more comprehensive, such as the Minnesota test devised by Schuell (1965).

If the patient has severe loss of comprehension, the therapist may use the Raven's Progressive Matrices, which do not demand understanding of verbal instructions, yet assess the basic intellectual deficit (Leche 1974). In addition, the therapist observes the breathing pattern of the patient, phonation, functioning of the lips and soft palate, and prosodic features such as speed, intonation and rhythm. In cases of dysarthria, she examines the components of speech which are causing slurring of consonants, and disturbances of rhythm, stress, intonation and speed of delivery. The ward sister could usefully assign a nurse to accompany the speech therapist, to observe an assessment, if the patient has no objection.

The main disadvantage of formal tests is that they discover nothing about what the patient does in his attempts to circumvent his verbal impairment, in his usual environment. Sometimes, when a patient shows no response to a test situation, he responds normally when in a spontaneous or natural situation. Such tests also fail to take into account that aphasic patients use gesture to communicate, or the time factor. For example, the patient may have intact speech, but needs time to use it, especially if the task set is very specific. In addition, these tests appear to be somewhat insensitive to either minimal or gross impairment. They are often more a measure of potential, than of actual language use. The nurse however, needs to know about the ability of the patient to function linguistically in his current environment. Consequently, a functional communica-nurse, however, needs to know about the ability of the patient to function lin-introduced separately, or in conjunction with the testing carried out by the speech therapist. The first profile should be compiled as soon as the patient recovers his physiological equilibrium, and this will form a base-line of information for future assessments. Such a profile (adapted from Taylor 1965), is shown in Table 115.

The rating assigned to the patient should take into account the following:

1 Speed of the patient's performance.

2 Accuracy of his response.

3 Consistency of his replies.

4 Extent of his voluntary control without the benefit of external cues.

5 Any compensatory function for the behaviour, e.g. pointing instead of speaking, which may be adequate, but not normal.

A functional profile offers an immediate picture of what the patient is capable of doing, and also serves as a record of achievement which can be used to motivate him in the weeks to come. A functional assessment may detect a subtle impairment in numerical concepts or arithmetic processes, or the slightest reduction in reading or writing skills. This may be important if the patient is eager to return to work. Such patients should be given a thorough functional evaluation, in an effort to prevent failing in an attempt to resume employment (Anderson 1970).

Management of therapy

Basic approaches in the treatment of aphasia

The principles of treatment determine the methods for language reorganization after the stroke, and involve other associated areas of the brain that they may restore function, and then use these or other residual powers to compensate for any deficit, and to acquire language (Leche 1974).

Table 15 Functional communication evaluation profile (adapted from Taylor 1965)

	Score 0-10	10-20	20-30	30-40	40-50	50-60	60-70	70-80	80-90	90-100	Percentage
Movement											Ability to imitate oral movement
											Attempt to communicate
											Ability to say 'yes' or 'no'
											Indicating floor in a lift
											Use of gestures
Speaking											Saying greetings
											Saying own name
											Saying nouns
											Saying verbs
											Saying noun-verb combinations
											Saying phrases (non-automatic)
											Giving directions
											Speaking on telephone
											Saying short complete sentences
											Saying long complete sentences
Understanding											Awareness of environment
											Awareness of emotional voice tone
											Understanding of own name
											Awareness of speech
											Recognition of family names
											Recognition of names of familiar objects
											Understanding action verbs
											Understanding gestured directions
											Understanding verbal directions
											Understanding conversation with one person
											Understanding short television programmes
											Understanding conversation with two people
											Understanding films or plays
											Understanding complicated verbal directions
											Understanding rapid complex conversation
Reading											Reading single words
											Reading post-card
											Reading street signs
											Reading newspaper headlines
											Reading letters
											Reading newspaper articles
											Reading magazines
											Reading books
Other											Writing name
											Time orientation
											Copying ability
											Writing from dictation
											Handling and describing money
											Using writing in lieu of speech
											Calculation ability

Plot premorbid ability in blue ink, present ability in red ink, and re-evaluation in another colour.

Taylor (1964b) identifies three basic approaches to the treatment of aphasia which incorporate these basic principles. She calls these stimulation, programmed instruction and socialization approaches.

Stimulation approach   The aim of stimulation therapy is maximal recovery of language function within the framework of the patient's needs. The environment is structured so that the patient is given every opportunity to communicate. This will help, through producing the cortical integration of stimulus and response necessary for language. It does not necessitate new learning, or the acquisition of a new vocabulary. Schuell et al. (1964) claim that the role to be adopted in this kind of situation should be that of communicator, not teacher. The therapist or nurse does not attempt to teach the patient sounds or words; rather she attempts to stimulate disrupted language processes to function as well as they can.

The carer should avoid using questions which demand a simple 'yes' or 'no' answer from the patient, such as, 'are you thirsty?' Rather more should be demanded, by asking questions which the patient completes with words that fit in with his everyday life. For example, to the question, 'what would you like to drink?', the patient has to apply an appropriate word, such as tea, coffee or milk. More patients have some ability to do this than is initially apparent, but often anxiety and tension inhibit performance.

The amount of stimulation a patient seeks or needs will vary with their normal life circumstances. For instance, Leche (1974) claims that a highly intelligent patient will be more severely handicapped than a less intelligent one with a comparable aphasic disorder. A professional man requires a much greater ability to cope with abstract thought processes than a labourer, who can mainly rely on more stereotyped responses. A bank manager, for example, is less likely to be able to return to his former employment, although his speech may have reached a level comparable to aphasia in a farmer which might be no longer apparent.

Programmed instruction approach The programmed instruction approach views language rehabilitation as more of an educative process, and uses operant conditioning techniques, drawn from theories of learning and psycholinguistic analyses, to guide the content and order of the presentation of linguistic thought (Holland 1970).

Programmed instruction is based on a belief that there are several separate stages of learning, including recognition, imitation, repetition and selection from a store of learned responses. This type of approach has been claimed as being particularly successful in expressive aphasics. Programmed instruction comes in various forms, including videotape (Hatfield 1971).

Socialization approach This type of approach demands flexibility in the therapeutic environment, and in the attitudes of staff. Group games or singing sessions act to release tensions, and encourage the patient to contribute in his own time, because no one is sitting next to him, awaiting his reply.

Disadvantages of group treatment include the difficulty of giving individual attention, the risk that some patients could become dominant over those who lack initiative, and the pace of the group, which may not suit all its members.

Basic principles in the treatment of dysarthria

Following the onset of dysarthria, specific exercises can be prescribed for the affected organs. These are designed to improve the range, mobility and coordination of movements concerned with respiration, phonation, resonance and articulation. Light brushing of the tip of the tongue, or applying ice, before therapy begins, helps the patient achieve some coordination of the oral musculature.

The nurse as a therapist and coordinator

An essential feature of any communication, especially any conversation, is that it is a two-way process. There must be someone to speak and, more importantly, someone to listen. Without someone to listen to him, a patient feels ignored, and sinks into linguistic isolation, even in a busy ward.

At home, there is a serious risk that the family, as well as the patient, can become isolated. Visitors may stop coming to the house because of the boredom, frustration or embarrassment which may result from trying to communicate with the patient. Even health professionals vary considerably in their ability to cope when compelled into a social situation with aphasic patients. They may attempt to resolve their discomfort, which could be interpreted as professionally unacceptable, by erecting a barrier of professionalism between themselves and the patient, which can disrupt a congenial therapeutic environment.

Professional infallibility is a factor implicit in all who wear uniforms or similar badges of status, which can act as a barrier between human beings. Some people continue to wear an invisible uniform after work is over, and conduct their personal relationships in a similar vein. Consequently, however well intentioned they may be, not all health personnel, family members or volunteers can work effectively with aphasic stroke patients. Participants who will be critical to the patient's progress should be selected with care. Seniority in a ward, or the closeness of a relationship at home, do not make selection automatic. A junior nurse may be more effective than a ward sister, or a daughter may be able to give more help to her father than his wife. This demands a certain amount of humility from those with natural authority, as well as immense skill on the part of the nurse in assessing and constructing the right therapeutic relationships for the patient, without promoting an atmosphere of guilt and inadequacy.

Support for the aphasic patient and his family should not be dependent solely on his need for physical care. A patient who cannot read, or understand the radio, may spend many aimless hours watching television. His family can become distressed as they find their lives increasingly revolving around the patient's inability or unwillingness to communicate and socialize. The whole situation might become too much for them. An occasional visit by a district nurse or health visitor may be all the support that a lonely spouse might need.

In spite of his limitations, the person who has suffered a stroke is still an intelligent, sensitive human being, with an awareness of the attitudes of those around him (McCartney 1974). The patient can learn far more about his situation from the non-verbal presentations of the nurse, than from a long verbal dissertation about his condition. However, it is still necessary that both patient and family understand what aphasia is, and why he does not understand all that is being said to him, or why he cannot express himself. Otherwise, the fear that he is 'losing his mind' may cause a panic in both the patient and his relatives (Kurasik and Sutton 1969). Not understanding what aphasia is can lead to a well-meaning relative beginning to anticipate the needs of the patient, and speaking for him when visitors call or in similar social situations. This deprives the patient of the opportunity to practise speaking, experiment, cope with his errors and gain confidence. He will lose motivation for improvement, which loss can manifest itself in the frequent use of phrases such as 'can't say' and 'don't know'. The more articulate, or socially dominant, the relative is, the more likely it is that he or she will assume such authority over the patient, unless the nurse can tactfully draw the attention of those concerned to what is happening.

Equally counterproductive is a situation which bombards the patient with demands for speech. If he can understand speech, it can become tiresome for him to be given language tests which appear childish, and he may simply choose to ignore them. If he has difficulty in comprehension, unstructured, haphazard attempts at therapy may confuse and demoralize. Nurses should not attempt therapy with the patient as they go about their other duties. The nurse's sense of urgency for a reply will communicate itself to the patient, and the results of his attempts to hurry with an answer to the nurse's intervention may embarrass him into silence. One or two short, but productive sessions each day will accomplish more, and reduce the anxiety and frustration associated with constant badgering. This does not mean that the nurse should not talk to the patient while performing nursing tasks, rather that normal conversation should not be presented as a form of therapy. If the patient cannot, or does not, communicate a need, it is easy for an assumption to be made that the need is reduced or absent, when in fact it may have become intensified.

At home, the patient should be allowed to attempt activities commensurate with his previous role in the family, providing it does not put his welfare, or that of the family, at risk. Whether in hospital or at home, a part of the patient's day should be set aside for work on speech, writing, reading, and also listening. Such daily schedules should be adhered to as consistently as possible, because aphasic stroke patients need to be able to anticipate what is going to happen. The external cues which the patient uses in hospital in order to anticipate events will be replaced by new ones when he is discharged. The family should be warned that he will need time to adjust, and have new schedules made out, which provide a framework for establishing new, appropriate cues to help his social behaviour. The patient's reliance on non-verbal cues should not be underestimated. His reliance on external cues can be tested in the following way. Take the patient to a quiet part of the room or ward where there are no distractions, and place a number of objects, of roughly the same size, in front of him. If one of these objects is a pencil, instruct him to pick it up. Avoid looking or even glancing at the pencil, before or during the instruction, and watch the patient's response. Did he look at the pencil and pick it up, or did he look into your face to seek further clues as to what he should do? He may be relying on the direction of the gaze of the speaker, rather than understanding the words.

Therapy should start at a level at which the patient is able to make a successful response. According to Schuell et al. (1964), auditory stimulation is the most effective therapeutic process to assist the aphasic in recovering language. Through this medium, they claim, the patient improves not only in his ability to understand, but also in his ability to talk, and read and write as well.

Hirschberg et al. (1976), advising on speech therapy sessions, say that relatives and staff should not expect dramatic changes in the patient's language function simply because he is receiving speech therapy. Improvement may be good 2-3 months after stroke, but it will become less striking thereafter. It might help to save any notes or other samples of work that the patient has done, so that he can compare them with future work. Constant reassurance and references to concrete signs of progress are necessary. The use of phrases such as, 'don't worry', or 'you'll be alright', without any accompanying explanatory context, could be interpreted by the patient as avoidance phrases, and lead him to feel that he is a hopeless case.

Hirschberg et al. (1976) suggest that speech-therapy sessions should follow a constant format, along the following lines:

1   Each session should begin with an easy task which the patient can do.
2   It should take place in a relaxed atmosphere.
3   Material previously covered should be reviewed.
4   If the patient copes with the review, new material should be offered that is interesting and relevant to the patient's circumstances.
5   The patient's attention should be drawn to his successes.
6   If he shows signs of fatigue the session should be stopped.

The speech therapist can give advice on how nursing staff might cope with a patient's language idiosyncracies. For example, a patient with receptive or fluent aphasia may respond more readily to a form of sentence construction which reflects his fluency. Rapid speech may allow some words to get across the comprehension barrier. Patients with expressive aphasia may respond to verbal cueing. For example, if asked to say 'pen' the patient may say nothing, but when the 'p' sound is made while the nurse is pointing to the object, he might be able to complete the sound by saying 'pen'.

Scrabble could be used as a therapeutic game for a patient who has difficulty speaking but whose comprehension is good.

Non-verbal techniques can be used to support verbal instructions. The nurse should demonstrate to the patient what is wanted of him, then touch the part of the body which he should move, and give the verbal command simultaneously. The expressive aphasic patient may prefer to be addressed in simple straightforward sentences, of single subject, verb, object construction, e.g. 'please sit on the chair'.

When practising writing, the patient might find it easier to use a pencil or felt-tip pen, rather than a ball-point pen. A ball-point pen is less easy to handle, because it needs to be held more vertically than a pencil. This demands more skill and effort to sustain, and the muscles of the hand tire more easily. Writing paper should be firmly attached to a hard surface, and be placed at a convenient height and reach. The patient might begin by copying his name and address, and then move on to more ambitious phrases and sentences.

The situation or circumstances of each aphasic stroke patient will be individual to him, and consequently every possible idiosyncratic detail cannot be discussed here. Some of the wide variety of terms used in language dysfunction are defined in the glossary at the end of the book. However, there are several points which a nurse should remember when helping any aphasic patient, in hospital or at home. These can be summarized as follows:

1 Do not shout at the patient; he is not deaf, speak to him in the normal way.

2 Speak slowly and clearly, but not childishly, or to the extent that he feels you are talking down to him.

3 Treat him as an adult; never talk about him with others in his presence, even if his comprehension is limited.

4 Present things to him in his visual field.

5 Be aware that his concentration may only last 5 minutes; so be prepared to change the task.

6 Try to make the work related to his own needs and interests.

7 Encourage any form of communication, whether it is by gesture, writing or speech.

8 Admit a lack of understanding; there is nothing more frustrating than a nurse who pretends she understands.

9 Try to think of the patient's ability and not his disability; try not to get upset if he swears.

10 Do not hurry him, or show signs of impatience.

11 The order of presentation of work to the patient is not as important as trying to end the session on a high note.

12 Try and work towards an agreed goal, no matter how small.

References

Adams, G F (1974) Cerebral Vascular Disability and the Ageing Brain, Churchill Livingstone

Adams, G F and Hurwitz, J (1963) Mental barriers to recovery from stroke, Lancet, (ii): 523-537

Altmann, N W (1972) Understanding your patient's emotions, Journal of Practical Nursing, 22: 22-25

Anderson, T P (1970) Management of completed stroke, Oklahoma State Medical Journal, 63: 403-411

Anderson, T P, Bourestrom, N, Greenberg, F R and Hilyard, V G (1974) Predictive factors in stroke rehabilitation, Archives of Physical Medicine and Rehabilitation, 55: 545-553

Baleman, F (1890) On Aphasia — A Loss of Speech and Localization of the Faculty of Articulate Language, 2nd edition, Churchill

Basso, A, Faglione, P and Vignolo, L (1975) Etude controlée de la rééducation du langage dans l'aphasie — comparaison entre aphasiques traités et non traités, Revue Neurologique, 131: 607

Bastian, H D (1880) The Brain as an Organ of the Mind, Kegan Paul, French, Trubner & Co

Benton, A L (1964) Contributions to aphasia before Broca, Cortex, 1: 314-327

Benton, A L and Joynt, R J (1960) Early description of aphasia, Archives of Neurology, 3: 205-222

Blondis, M N and Jackson, B E (1977) Non-verbal Communication with Patients — Back to the Human Touch, J Wiley & Sons

Bright, R (1972) Music in Geriatric Care, Angus & Robertson

Broca, P (1861a) Remarques sur le siège de la faculté du langage articulé suivies d'une observation d'aphémie (perte de la parole), Bulletin de la Société Anatomique de Paris, XXVI: 2me série, August: 331

Brocklehurst, J C , Andrews, K, Richards, B and Laycock, P J (1978) How much physical therapy for patients with stroke? British Medical Journal, 1: 1307-1310

Brust, J, Schafer, S, Richter, R, and Bruun, B (1976) Aphasia in acute stroke, Stroke, 7: 167

Buck, McKenzie (1970) Dysphasia — the patient, his family and the nurse, Cardiovascular Nursing, 6 (5): 51-56

Butterfield, E and Zangwill, O (1946) Re-education in aphasia — a review of seventy cases, Journal of Neurology, Neurosurgery and Psychiatry, 9: 75-79

Cameron, C (1973) A Different Drum, Prentice Hall

Charcot, J M and Pitres, A (1883) Etude critique et clinique de la localization matrices, F Alcan

Christie, D and Lawrence, L (1978) Patients and hospitals — a study of the attitudes of stroke patients, Social Science and Medicine, 12: 49-51

Conrad, K (1954) New problems of aphasia, Brain, 77: 491-501

Critchley, McDonald (1970) Aphasiology and Other Aspects, Edward Arnold

Dahlberg, C and Jaffee, J (1977) Stroke — A Physician's Personal Account, W. Norton

De Reuk, A V S and O'Connor, M (1964) Disorders of Language — Ciba Foundation Symposium, Little, Brown & Co

DeVito, J (1970) Psychology of Speech and Language, Random House

Ekmann, P and Frieson, W V (1975) Unmasking the Face, Prentice Hall

Gardner, H, Albert, M L and Weintraubs, S (1975) Comprehending a word — the influence of speed and redundancy on auditory comprehension in aphasia, Cortex, 11: 155-162

Garraway, W M, Walton, M S, Akhtar, A J and Prescott, R J (1980) The use of health and social services in the management of stroke in the community — results from a controlled trial, Age and Ageing, 10: 95-104

Gazzaniga, M S and Sperry, R W (1967) Language after section of the cerebral commisures, Brain, 90: 131-148

Geschwind, N (1965) Disconnexion syndromes in animals and man, Brain, 88: 237 and 585-644

Geschwind, N (1970a) The clinical syndromes of cortical connections, in D Williams (Editor) Modern Trends in Neurology, Volume 5, Butterworths

Geschwind, N (1970b) The organisation of language and the brain, Science 170: 940-944

Geschwind, N (1974) Selected Papers on Language and the Brain, Volume XVI, D Reidel

Godfrey, C and Douglas, E (1959) The recovery process in aphasia, Canadian Medical Association Journal, 80: 618

Goldstein, K (1939) The Organism, American Book Co

Gough, D and Powell, C (1978a) Aphasia and the nurse — part 1, Nursing Mirror, 147 (5): 28-29

Gough, D and Powell, C (1978b) Aphasia and the nurse — part 2, Nursing Mirror, 147 (6): 29-30

Gowers, W R (1885) Diseases of the Brain, J & A Churchill

Hagen, C (1973) Communication abilities in hemiplegia — effect of speech therapy, Archives of Physical Medicine and Rehabilitation, 54: 454

Hatfield, F M (1971) Some uses of videotape recording in language rehabilitation after brain damage, Medical and Biological Illustrations, 21 (3): 166-171

Head, H (1926) Aphasia and Kindred Disorders of Speech, 2 volumes, McMillan

Hebb, D O (1961) The Organization of Behaviour, J Wiley & Sons

Hirschberg, C C, Lewis, L and Vaughan, P (1976) Rehabilitation, J B Lippincott

Holland, A L (1970) Case studies in aphasia rehabilitation using programmed instruction, Journal of Speech and Hearing, 35: 377-390

Hunt, T (1851) A case of amnesia, American Journal of Insanity, 7: 358

Hurwitz, L J and Adams, G F (1972) Rehabilitation of hemiplegia — indices of assessment and prognosis, British Medical Journal, 1: 94-98

Jackson Hughlings, J (1931) The Selected Writings, Volume 2 — Speech, Hodder & Stoughton

Jakobson, R and Halle, M (1956) Fundamentals of Language, Mouton

Kenin, M and Swisher, L (1972) A study of the pattern of recovery in aphasia, Cortex, 8: 56

Kersetz, A and McCabe, P (1977) Recovery patterns and prognosis in aphasia, Brain, 100: 1-18

Kerschensteiner, M, Poeck, K and Brunner, E (1972) The fluency-non fluency dimension in the classification of aphasic speech, Cortex, 8: 233

Knapp, M E (1959) Problems in rehabilitation of the hemiplegic patient, Journal of the American Medical Association, 169: 224-229

Kurasik, S and Sutton, B B (1969) Management of the hemiplegic stroke patient, Journal of American Geriatrics, 17: 701-709

Kussmaul, A (1877) Die Störungen der Sprache, F C W Vogel

Leche, P M (1974) The speech therapist and hemiplegia, Physiotherapy, 60 (11): 346-349

Licht, S (1975) A brief history of stroke and its rehabilitation, in Licht, S (ed) Stroke and its rehabilitation, Licht, E

Luria, A R (1970) Traumatic aphasia — its syndromes, psychology and treatment, Mouton

Laria, A R, Tsretskova, L S and Futer, D S (1965) Aphasia in a composer, Journal of Neurological Sciences, 2: 288-292

McCartney, V C (1974) Rehabilitation and dignity for the stroke patient, Nursing Clinics of North America, 9: 693-701

Marie, P (1906) Révision de la question de l'aphasie — la troisième convolution frontale gauche ne joue aucun rôle spécial dans la fonction du langage, Semaine Médicale, 26: 241-247

Marie, P (1922) Étude clinique sur les modalités des dissociations dans lésion encephaliques, Revue Neurologique, 29: 14

Meikle, M (1981) Listen, I want to tell you something, Nursing Times, 77, Aug: supplement 10-14

Meikle, M, Wechsler, E, Tupper, A, Benenson, M, Butler, J, Mulhall, D and Stern, G (1979) Comparative trial of volunteer and professional treatments of aphasia after stroke, British Medical Journal, 2: 87-89

Mills, C (1904) Aphasia and the central zones of speech, American Journal of Medical Science, 16: 375-377

Mitchell, J (1958) Speech and language impairment in the older patient, Geriatrics, 13: 467-476

Moss, C (1972) Recovery in Aphasia — The Aftermath of My Stroke, University of Illinois Press

Nichol, P J R (1971) Rehabilitation Medicine, Butterworths

208   Nursing Care of the Hemiplegic Stroke Patient

Osgood, C E and Miron, M S (1970) Approaches in the Study of Aphasia — A Report on an Interdisciplinary Conference on Aphasia, University of Illinois Press

Patrick, G (1973) Forgotten patients on the medical ward, The Canadian Nurse, 68: (3): 27-31

Patterson, A (1971) The speech therapist's role in stroke rehabilitation, Modern Geriatrics, 1: 403-407

Penfield, W and Roberts, L (1959) Speech and Brain Mechanisms, Princeton University Press

Perrine, G (1971) Needs met and unmet, American Journal of Nursing, 71: 9128-2133

Policoff, L D (1970) The philosophy of stroke rehabilitation, Geriatrics, 25: 97-100

Quinting, G G (1971) Hesitation Phenomena in Adult Aphasia and Normal Speech, Mouton

Riese, W (1947) The early history of aphasia, Bulletin of Medical History, 21: 322

Roaf, R and Hodkinson, L J (1977) The Paralysed Patient, Blackwell Scientific Publications

Rolnick, M and Hoops, H R (1969) Aphasia as seen by the aphasic, Journal of Speech and Hearing, 34: 49-53

Rosenthal, A M (1971) Home management of the hemiplegic patient, American Family Physician, 3: 114-119

Salley, C M and Murphey, G (1960) Development of the Perceptual World, Basic Books

Sarno, M T (1976) The status of recovery in aphasia, in Y Lebrun and R Hoops (Editors) Recovery in Aphasics — Neurolinguistics, Swets & Zeitlinger

Savage, B J and Widdowson, T (1974) Revising the use of nursing resources, Nursing Times, 70: 1372-1374

Schow, R L, Christensen, J M, Hutchinson, J M and Nerbonne, M A (1978) Communication Disorders of the Aged — A Guide for Health Professionals, University Park Press, Baltimore

Schuell, H (1965) The Minnesota Test for Differential Diagnosis of Aphasia, University of Minnesota Press

Schuell, H, Jenkins, J J and Jimenez-Pablon, E (1964) Aphasia in Adults — Diagnosis, Prognosis and Therapy, Hoeber Medical Division

Schwab, J J (1972) Emotional considerations in stroke, New York State Medical Journal, 72: 2877-2880

Sies, L F (editor) (1974) Aphasia Theory and Therapy — Selected Lectures and Papers of Hildred Schuell, Macmillan Press

Smith, A (1971) Objective indices of severity of chronic aphasia in stroke patients, Journal of Speech and Hearing, 36: 167-207

Taylor, M L (1964a) Linguistic considerations of the verbal behaviour of the brain in a damaged adult, The Linguistic Reporter, 6 (3): 1

Taylor, M L (1964b) Language therapy, in H G Burr (Editor) The Aphasic Patient — Evaluation and Rehabilitation, Wayside Press

Taylor, M L (1965) Measurement of functional evaluation in aphasia, Archives of Physical Medicine and Rehabilitation, 46: 101-107

Vignolo, L A (1964) Evolution of aphasia and language rehabilitation — a retrospective exploratory study, Cortex, 1: 344-367

Wagenaar, E, Snow, C and Prins, R (1975) Spontaneous speech of aphasic patients — a psycholinguistic approach, Brain Language, 2: 281

Weddell, J M and Beresford, S A A (1979) Planning for Stroke Patients, HMSO

Weisenberg, T and McBride, W (1964) Aphasia — A Clinical and Psychological Study, Hofner

Wepman, J M (1951) Recovery from Aphasia, Ronald Press

Wernicke, C (1874) Der Aphasische Symptomen Komplex, Taschen

Whittet, M M (1971) Rehabilitation of the stroke patient, Rehabilitation, 79: 13-15

World Health Organisation (1971b) Stroke — treatment, rehabilitation and prevention, WHO Chronicle, 25, Oct: 466-469

Wulf, H (1973) Aphasia — My World Alone, Wayne State University Press

Zangwill, O (1964) The current status of cerebral dominance — a research publication for the Association for Research, Nervous and Mental Diseases (Baltimore), 42: 103-118

CHAPTER 9

NURSING MANAGEMENT OF
SPIRITUAL COMFORT

Why me?
No one can know what I feel like now!
But my mother was always such a kind, caring person!
There aren't words to describe it!
They (the doctors) just pass by my bed — they don't care!
I feel like a baby!
What have I to live for?
The nurses just didn't see me as a human being!
What's going to happen? We were so looking forward to our retirement!
Am I going to be like this for twenty years?
What's the purpose of it all?
If that ever happened to me, I think I'd kill myself!
I suppose if there is a life after death he's bought his ticket!
My father would be better off dead!
What good am I to anyone now?

These are quotes from patients, relatives and staff, who were attempting to adjust spiritually to the presence of stroke in their lives. While not mentioning 'God', they were seeking to express their innermost feelings, and needed to share their distress with another human being (in this case the author, an almost total stranger). In other words, they were looking for an explanation for a situation which they did not understand. Those suffering or sharing a catastrophe often unwittingly look for support. However, although it may be the nurse who is asked to provide such support, a perusal of nursing literature or curriculae will show that the nurse is often ill prepared to adopt the role of spiritual comforter.

McGilloway and Donnelly (1977) claim that:

> . . . emphasis is still placed upon the obligation to respect the religious beliefs of the patient at times of death and birth, and whenever important moral issues, for example, euthanasia, sterilisation and transplantation, arise. But it is tempting to say that many of us do not yet appreciate, or perhaps overlook, the importance of the spiritual needs of the ordinary ill person in the hospital bed. We are certainly uninformed.

It would appear that the socialization process in nursing ill prepares the learner for anything more than superficial contact between herself and her patient. It tends to militate against a learning *with* her patients. Sitting and talking to patients is still actively discouraged on some wards, and learners are often told that they should not get emotionally involved with their patients, because a process of detachment is deemed essential for objective care and treatment. The hospital style of care can create loneliness in both staff and patients, and Wilson (1971) claims that such loneliness is usually seen as simply another problem to be solved, rather than as a symptom of possible loss of vision of the whole enterprise. The rigidity of hospital relationships can act as a barrier between staff and patients. Against such a trend, it might be argued that the student nurse or doctor needs to learn, not to avoid involvement with the patient; she needs, rather, to discipline such involvement.

The religious and military background of nursing encourages the nurse to forget herself, through orientation and service to other people. It encourages her to suppress her human beingness, the very thing that reaches out to others. The uniform, the hierarchical structure of nursing, and the expectations of others, can lead to the nurse adopting a persona or mask which she can come to identify as herself. Thus, she can lose sight of her real self, which should be growing up within her as she comes to grips with her own and her patient's life problems.

Finally, both patient and nurse find themselves in an increasingly technocratic society. In such an environment, there is a risk of an overgrowth of intellectual concerns, without a counterdevelopment of the emotional and spiritual, with the result that all concerned may become lessened as human beings.

This is possibly the most important, and the most difficult, chapter of this book on the care of the stroke patient, because it is in this area, more than any other, that the nurse has to sustain the giving of herself. The care process which she offers may or may not be validated by physical or biochemical results, and the relationship alone may have to remain paramount as the motivating force for both participants. The tragedy of stroke is not simply something to be overcome in physical terms; rather it is an experience to be understood by the nurse as well as the patient and, if faced responsibly, both can emerge as healthier human beings, spiritually if not physically.

This chapter will ask questions — the reader will provide the answers. It adopts the perspective that the nurse's role in spiritual comfort lies in more than offering the correct diet, or arranging the relevant religious sacrament; rather hers is the role of an enabler. She helps the patient, the relatives and the other staff to come to terms with the reality of human fragility and mortality. This chapter will question attitudes to suffering, and the redemptive status of suffering. It will also examine the role which formal religious practices and their ministers may play, particularly in a hospital environment. This will be a strictly personal point of view, and other nurses may agree or disagree with what is written, according to their own beliefs. Nevertheless, the cries for help from stroke patients and their families, quoted at the beginning of this chapter, demand that a discussion takes place.

Religion and mystical experience

The word 'religion', like the word 'God', is ambiguous. It has different meanings for different people. For example, American Indians do not pray to a god, but to a principle existing in all created life, and which they believe is accessible and responsive to man.

Many people, especially in the Western world, regard religion as a matter of belief in a certain system of theological doctrines. Isherwood (1970) claims that the trouble with such doctrines is that their adherents, when of limited knowledge and over-suggestibility to authority, tend to suppose themselves to be in possession, not merely of a ray of light, but of the whole truth. Their church is the 'one true fold', its canon is closed and there is nothing more to be discussed. She writes that, 'they have narrowed down the Universe to the limits of their own understanding . . . always the sectarian believes that all truth is contained in his own little pool.'

For purposes of discussion it is useful to distinguish between a religion which consists of a system of doctrinal teachings to be believed, and religion as inner experience, sometimes called 'mysticism'. Such a distinction is relevant to nursing, if one accepts that true religion does not require one to believe; rather it requires one to become. It is a state to be attained, rather than a set of proportions to be accepted. Therefore, in her unselfishness, concern and sensitivity towards others, the nurse is in fact more 'religious' than many so-called staunch believers. The act of nursing takes from all ideologies. The word religion itself is derived from the Latin word ligare, meaning 'to bind together'.

A survey of the world religions cannot be pursued here, and their philosophies and obligations are well documented elsewhere (e.g. Nigosian 1975). Whether monotheistic or pluralistic, it is the meaning which the religious belief holds for the patient which is important. Consequently, how the nurse might facilitate such a belief in a patient becomes an integral part of the nursing care plan. This is particularly important for the stroke patient, who sees death as imminent, or who faces a life-long struggle to come to terms with his disability. The language of the distress of the soul is sometimes known as 'existentialism', because it deals with such themes as anxiety, guilt, despair, loneliness and self-doubt.

Monotheism is the belief that there is only one Supreme Being, and a monotheistic faith, such as Christianity, finds expression in prayers, commandments, parables, psalms and other Biblical teachings, which have been philosophically elaborated and defined through the long history of Christian thought (Hicks 1963). However, atheists (non-believers) and agnostics (don't knows) can and do philosophize about religion and, therefore, should not be ignored.

Pluralistic religions, such as Hinduism, believe in the existence of more than one god, each god having a specific function. Some believe that religion is what a person does with his solitude. Such aspirants seek retreat through yoga or transcendental meditation. Eastern religions claim that the highest form of religion one can know is mystic experience, or illumination, a state known by many names, e.g. Nirvana. In the early 1960s, many young people used hallucinatory drugs such as LSD in an attempt to attain this state artificially.

All religions which include god-worship seek a total and unqualified response from their believers. According to Hicks (1963), the Christian concept of God is one conceived as the infinite, eternal, uncreated, personal reality, who has created all that exists, other than Himself, and who has revealed Himself to his creatures as holy and loving. This in itself implies retribution to those who go against His wishes.

It has been a persistent claim of those wholeheartedly committed to Christian discipleship that tragedy, though truly tragic, may be turned, through man's reaction, from a cause of despair and alienation from God to the fulfilment of God's loving purpose for the sufferer. A wider philosophy may complement such a philosophy. For example, Tillich (1951) claims that religion is the state of being grasped by an ultimate concern, which qualifies all other concerns as preliminary and which itself contains the answer to the question of the meaning of our life. Therefore, he claims that:

> God . . . is the name for that which concerns man ultimately. This does not mean that first there is a being called God, and then the demand that man should be ultimately concerned about him. It means that whatever concerns a man ultimately, becomes God for him, and conversely, it means that man can be concerned ultimately only about that which is God for him.

Instead of the word 'ultimate', it has been suggested that the word 'deep' or 'intense' should be substituted, because 'ultimate' does not admit of degrees, which affect all realms of human interest (Edwards 1972).

The Tillichian philosophy appears to overcome semantic differences of religious language and definition. It is this deep, intense, or ultimate concern which the nurse is seeking to discover in her patient, and to move along positive, healthy lines.

The concept of suffering

Suffering is an ill-applied word in modern society. We say a people 'suffers' from famine, a family 'suffers' from low income, or a country 'suffers' from inflation. Consequently, suffering is a word which by its personal, subjective nature, cannot be easily defined. Here it is used in the context of ill health and disability.

That suffering exists is usually accepted as fact by most people. Indeed, to be able to explain why suffering exists will not absolve its reality. Bowker (1970) claims that the problem is not that suffering exists, but why it affects some people and not others. 'Why me?' Sometimes obstacles breed strength of character, evoke great courage and unselfishness, produce extreme courage and moral steadfastness. However, as any nurse is well aware, the same obstacles can also lead to deep resentment, fear, selfishness and disintegration of character. Therefore, if what Hicks (1963) calls, 'the business of soulmaking', is worth all the toil and sorrow for patient and carer, there must be a belief in a future good, such as the existence of life after death. Bowker (1970) claims that discipleship in Christ actually involves suffering and, therefore, suffering is an important component of identification with Christianity, as a way of continually asserting and realizing Christ's victory.

In personal terms, for the nurse, this means avoiding all behaviour that might cause suffering to others, and taking effective action to relieve suffering. There is a similarity throughout all religions in their attitudes to suffering. For example, the Islamic attitude is that suffering, especially sickness, patiently endured, remits sins.

The word suffering implies that something is not completed, that it is unfinished; it is in some way not whole. A new wholeness has to be created by the integration of this struggle within, or against suffering, into growth towards a maturity which will give some illumination into the meaning of it all.

All those concerned with the patient seek for overt, concrete explanations for his and their own situation. This is, after all, not new. Thoughtful people of all ages, and throughout time, have wondered about life, and that special something which gives life significance, especially in the face of suffering. There is also a deep need to feel that how we live matters. Isherwood (1970) claims that it is psychologically and spiritually dangerous to attempt to meet these needs or answer these questions in terms of rigid and often debatable theology. After all, an image of a loving God may be difficult for a young stroke victim to retain. Through his experience, and thinking, his beliefs and thoughts of God and religion may change. It is the feeling between the nurse and the patient which may register, not the indoctrination of words; indeed the words 'God' or 'religion' might never be mentioned. When a patient demands from a nurse that she provide an answer to what he is suffering, and the nurse replies she cannot because there are many things she does not know, she is offering the patient the beginnings of humility in the face of ignorance. In the long term this may be more important than the information which he sought in the first instance. The role of the nurse, when faced with suffering, may not be to try to solve the problem intellectually, with reason or doctrine, but to try and raise the level of consciousness in the patient, relative or staff member, as a way for them to come to see things differently, and less gloomily, by talking it through. The problems of humanity are rarely solved by doctrine, but through regenerating what is positive in the attitudes of individuals.

A simple reliance on the redemptive status of suffering may act as a metaphysical form of barrier to the growth of the nurse and patient as individuals, through preventing the sharing of pleasant and unpleasant experiences.

The redemptive status of suffering   When I sit in the dentist's chair, I feel I am suffering, but I could not claim my suffering has any redemptive status. If I complain to my friends, they would dismiss my moaning with comments such as 'your teeth are old', or 'you should look after your teeth!'

If a 16 year old motor cyclist becomes permanently paralyzed in an accident, the neighbours of the family might be heard to say, 'how awful, but wasn't he always a bit of a tearaway?' But when a 6 year old child lies dying of cancer, or a young woman lies bedridden with rheumatoid arthritis, or a new-born baby is suddenly lost, what do we say?

Not all suffering has redemptive status, and there are different levels or strata of redemption. In the first two examples, the 'how' of the suffering is apparently explained, in that there is a reason for it. It may be seen as the inevitability of ageing, the neglect of the individual concerned or of others. In other instances, an hereditary or family trait may be supposed.

The 'how' may give indication to the 'why'. For example, if the stroke patient has had hypertension for several years, and his father died of stroke, then a stroke may be seen as being a somewhat inevitable pathological process in his ageing. If he had taken no steps to obtain a hypotensive agent, then the redemptive status of his suffering might be reduced even further. It is when one cannot apply any explanation in physical or psychological terms to the affliction, or when the 'how' is insufficient to explain the 'why', that human nature seeks metaphysical explanations, often through religious symbolism. There is a desire to call upon God when we feel we can no longer safely call upon ourselves, and our experiences.

The desire for a supernatural explanation will vary between individuals, races, religions and societies, because the redemptive status of suffering is dependent on socio-cultural norms. For example, self-inflicted suffering, undertaken on behalf of others, is respected as a sacrifice among many religious groups. Crucifixion for Christians and self-burning in Buddhism are symbolic of caring for human society. The Christian monk who practises self-flagellation, and the Hindu holy man who stands on one leg for 20 years, are both respected for the suffering or deformity which they inflict upon themselves in order to attain spiritual ascendancy. Therefore, the redemptive status of self-inflicted suffering may depend on what personal reward the individual might be seen as hoping to attain, by others in his group. The attempted suicide often receives scant sympathy in hospital, especially if the nurse believes such an act is sinful, and that the patient was only seeking attention.

Consequently, while individual persons will attempt to explain what is outside their experience in terms of redemptive suffering, no two individuals will perceive the situation in exactly the same way. A nurse and patient of the same religious persuasion may regard the patient's suffering in broadly the same way, but they may differ regarding the intensity of the suffering, or the extent of its redemptive status. The nurse, as well as the patient, is a product of her own society and its cultural and religious norms.

The ethic, 'the religious beliefs of the patient shall be respected', removes from the nurse the task of being evangelical. This means that her service to the patient does not have to depend upon her *own* beliefs, though these will be implicit in her service. It does not mean that the nurse should diminish the value of her own belief, only that proselytizing under the cloak of humanitarianism is unhealthy. To expound the redemptive status of suffering within close theological doctrine may result in the development of fatalism, out of a sense of powerlessness. Fatalism can, in turn, result in feelings of passivity, stagnation and impotence. The nurse can give the patient's existential being a positive and dynamic, rather than passive, direction, by understanding and working with the patient within the therapeutic process, rather than attempting either to struggle against the reality of stroke, or imposing external explanations. The notion of service has to retain its content of partnership and critical responsibility. Giving alone may hurt and divide, because it emphasizes the separation between the giver and the receiver, between the healthy and the sick (Wilson 1971). Sharing will be the most likely and persistent healer.

Sharing and spiritual dependency

Communication in hospital centres around the communication of information, but both staff and patients are constantly communicating aspects of themselves to each other. While nurse educationalists emphasize the need to keep a patient informed regarding his illness, nevertheless, a fully informed patient may be starving from lack of communication with his fellow human beings. Gabo (1959) claims that specialization in hospital life leads to fragmentation, and a loss of vision in the healing process as a whole. The consequence could be that our care of the patient's life becomes limited by our interest in the function which he performs. If the function of the hospital is to give, implicit in the giving is the witholding. Control of information can, in turn, control the behaviour pattern of the patient. If he is not allowed to share the truth about his illness, he may be forced to live a lie, and he may then be unable to make anything of the situation (Wilson 1971). To experience and grow from his catastrophe, the stroke patient must not be denied the very material he needs to answer the question, 'what ought I now to become?'

Fragmentation of function, as exemplified in task-orientated nursing, can erect a barrier to communication between the giver and receiver, or the nurse and the patient.

There may sometimes be conflict between staff, and between relatives, about what the patient should or should not be told, and when the best time for telling might be. It is important that any such conflict should be borne by the right people. For example, a learner should not be left to cope with a patient who asks if he is going to die, or have another stroke, because the doctor and the ward sister differ in their approach to telling the truth.

The word 'patient' denotes one who is passive and who submits to others. The questioning patient is sometimes classed by nursing staff as awkward. The fear of victimization is real and, alas, frequently justified. The 'good' patient is one who does as he is asked, and who fits into the hierarchical organization of the ward. Nurses feel comfortable with such patients, and class them as popular (Stockwell 1972).

The nurse in charge feels comfortable with the patient who belongs to a particular religious group, especially one where the religious obligations do not conflict with her role. For example, when an ill patient is a member of the Roman Catholic or Jewish faith, her obligations demand that she informs the priest or rabbi in order that specific sacraments can be fulfilled. The formality of this procedure fits neatly into her concept of the formal structures in the ward environment. If she is of the same religious persuasion as the patient, there need be even less hesitation in meeting or understanding the needs of the patient. If she is of a different faith, or the religious belief of the patient is less distinct, the situation may demand qualities which she finds difficult to reconcile within a formal structure. In other words, where formality exists in religious or spiritual matters, the nurse in charge tends to feel more comfortable, because she is aware of the parameters of her responsibility.

All ill people regress to some degree in terms of dependency. Indeed, may it not be necessary to regress in order to rebuild, particularly a shattered life? Illness or disability may present a creative opportunity for adaptation and growth. The experience of what life has to offer, whether good or bad, pleasant or unpleasant, should be seen as part of self-fulfilment. Experience should not be denied any individual; rather it should be controlled so the patient can be supported throughout.

Balint (1957) poses questions which face all nurses, namely how dependent should one let a patient become, and for how long? How much regression is permissible, and when? When should one push a patient into being responsible? Nurses frequently ask such questions in relation to physical regression and dependency. It is perhaps also necessary to ask similar questions in relation to spiritual dependency. If we regress physically and intellectually, can we not also regress spiritually? It may be possible that sick people who have lapsed from belief, return, in their illness or disability, to an infantile form of religion, just where they left it years before. It is difficult to define what impact a regressive physical state might have on the patient's spiritual dependency level. Wilson (1971) found that, of those among the hospital patients he surveyed who never attended church, 13.3% wanted their local minister to be told about their admission.

Pastoral advice, especially relating to the redemptive status of suffering, may perhaps serve to strengthen a passive role for the patient. It would seem important that the ministrations of the priest, vicar or nurse should not be used simply as another 'drug' by the patient; rather staff should insist on the patient being treated, and expecting to be treated, as a person with responsibility in maintaining his own physical and spiritual independence.

Finally, speaking about spiritual matters with a patient when he is ill prepared will not necessarily relieve his anxiety; it might actually cause it.

The role of the chaplain

In cases of self-doubt related to the provision of spiritual comfort, nurses are encouraged, in a standard manner, to turn to the chaplain for help and advice. McGilloway and Donnelly (1977) claim that:

> . . . the most important function, for the chaplain, is when he makes it possible for the patient to enter into a relationship with God, through ritual and other means. There are patients who look for rituals, for authority, for structural forms and objective beliefs, but there are those who are suspicious of rituals, who emphasise the 'personal' aspect of religion and prefer less structured organisation. Anyone sensitive to the feelings of those in their care will not ignore these differences.

As with other health care staff, the chaplain experiences conflict in his hospital work. Wilson (1971) claims that the chaplain is expected by the ward sister to give comfort to individual sick patients, but in reality he is not primarily interested in people because they are sick; rather he is interested in people who happen to be patients, not patients who happen to be people. The chaplain, of whatever religious persuasion, is not particularly interested in sickness, rather in a style of living, secular or spiritual, which is lived in sickness or health.

Nursing staff expect to see the chaplain busily visiting sick patients, but his work is primarily the work of prayer, rather than deed alone. Without the support of reflective contemplation, and prayer, he will feel his actions are shallow and without meaning. Although counselling of anxious and frightened patients or relatives is part of his role, he is also concerned in supporting their strengths as well as their weaknesses. Consequently, the chaplain has to reconcile what he wants to achieve in the hospital with the expectations of the staff and patients. In his survey, Wilson (1971) found that doctors tended to describe the chaplain's role in functional terms, and to assess it by their normal medical criteria of the patient's recovery. Patients and nurses, however, spoke of the chaplain in terms of friendship and personal qualities. Nevertheless, 80% of patients interviewed saw the chaplain's role in terms of taking services, prayers and other formal activities.

Situational factors also impinge on perspectives. McGilloway and Donnelly (1977) indicate that the chaplain deals with patients in contexts which are strongly charged with emotional and expressively symbolic significance, and which are considered particularly private to the patient himself. They claim that, just as discretion by all team members is a feature that is important in the total care of the patient, this also applies to the chaplain. They write that, 'in the performance of his duty, a fact may be revealed which may not be conveyed, even if important in the sense of health needs, to other members of the team'.

The chaplain as an individual contributes to his projected image. Some chaplains tend to call and see only their own parishioners, or church attenders, or only those of their own religious persuasion. Others speak to, or pray with, any patient. There are chaplains who, despite their sincerity, wear their ecclesiastical dress like a badge, and look decidedly uncomfortable in the role of universal comforter. The creed of the chaplain might dictate his behaviour, but his training or personality may not help him to fulfil the expectation of his creed, particularly in the hospital environment.

Nurses also receive very little help from their training, on how they might incorporate formal or informal spiritual care into their nursing plans. Learners may be given one or more talks or formal lectures by chaplains, usually during the introductory course, but are then left to learn through the example of other nurses. This presents a risk that the chaplain comes to be seen as someone who steps in at the point of the ward sister's weakness in dealing with spiritual comfort, or because he can speak of God, and she cannot.

Nurse training should make it possible for staff to learn to use the chaplain to deepen the quality of their own patient care, not to encourage him to take it out of their hands. Wilson (1971) claims that a nurse should be prepared to assume responsibility in spiritual matters. She should refer the patient's questions to another person only with the utmost caution, because confidences are difficult to share twice, and there is always a reason why one person is chosen, and not someone else. Therefore, it is part of the work of the nurse to give humane spiritual ministry when called upon to do so by the patient or relative, or even other staff members, despite any feelings of inadequacy. It is the ability to undertake such personal counsel and help which is the mark of both professional and personal maturity. It is no real answer to suggest that the patient calls in a chaplain, for he can help some, but not others. After all, spontaneity is distinctive of truly personal communication between human beings who recognize the value of each other. Many young nurses fail to respond, because they feel that they have not been *given* the authority to do so, though this failure is in conflict with what they feel as human beings. However, it is usually the young nurse who will be approached by the patient with problems, because the ward sister is remote, and always appears busy.

Ward sisters rarely invite the chaplain to help them with patient care. They tend to refer to him only if he is present on the ward for other purposes. Whether or not the ward sister approaches him for help may depend on his personal attributes, e.g. his age in relation to hers, and whether or not he is easy to get on with (Wilson 1971).

It may be likely that patients will accept chaplains from denominations other than their own for informal counselling, but not for formal services, such as the sacraments. Again, there is a degree of difference between churches, in that the authority of the Roman Catholic priest must be respected by one of his faith, regardless of personal preferences for him as a person. The help which a ward sister may request is often restricted to accepted religious activities. For example, all mainstream Christian churches play down the paranormal gifts of healing, such as faith healing or laying on of hands, with the consequence that the ward sister will be disinclined to seek help in this area.

There may be misunderstanding between the chaplain and the nurse in respect of a patient who is dying. It should be remembered that a heavily sedated patient is in no condition to receive formal or informal spiritual comfort from anyone. Nurses and doctors tend to see death within the framework of failure of their roles as givers. However, a chaplain will not believe that death is the worst thing that can happen to a person. He will not see his role only in terms of illness and death, and for the patient alone, but as a counsellor for relatives and staff. Yet chaplains do not normally have access to the medical records of ill patients, and are rarely invited to share in case conferences with staff.

Nurses in long-term care wards frequently have to act as spiritual comforters to their patients, because of the neglect of chaplains. Wilson (1971) found that patients over 60 years of age are less likely to be spoken to by clergymen than younger patients. Elderly patients relate their contact with the chaplain as being less close than that of younger patients. The older Roman Catholic patient was more likely to be visited than a patient of the Protestant faith. In addition, local ministers tended to visit more middle-class than working-class patients. That patients are not encouraged by staff to use the facility of the hospital chapel cannot be disputed. Only 8.8% of the large number of patients in Wilson's survey used the hospital chapel, and only 20% claimed that they were not inclined to do so anyway. The majority of those who would have liked to have attended services, but who did not go, gave a medical reason for non-attendance, such as the doctor's ward round. A little co-operation could prevent this happening.

When chaplains did talk to patients, Wilson found that casual remarks and general conversation accounted for 82% of conversations. Religious discussion occupied only 9.2% of the chaplain's time in the ward, counselling personal problems 4.8%, and formal sacraments 3.9%. There were no perceived differences between the sexes relating to what was discussed with the chaplain.

Chaplains spend far less time visiting long-stay wards. After being in hospital over 1 month, Wilson found that 43% of such patients had not been visited either by a hospital chaplain or their own minister. Yet it is in such wards that despair rather than hope may prevail.

The conclusion which the reader might reach from this discussion is that there is no one rule governing the provision of spiritual comfort to any patient. Judgement as to when to push forward, or when to hold back, comes not only from experience in nursing, but also from knowledge of the patient as a person. It would appear that the nurse could make more use of the hospital chaplain within her programme of care, and not restrict contact to when she feels she cannot cope, or when the patient requests help himself. When hospital chapel facilities are available, and the patient's clinical condition permits, more effort might be put into organizing his day in order that he might attend services, or enjoy a private visit. A radio or television service is invaluable for bedfast or housebound patients. Even if the patient is not able to concentrate, he can enjoy the atmosphere of the service. In hospitals, especially in long-term care wards, local choirs should not be restricted to performing at Christmas festivities. Stroke victims enjoy music like anyone else.

The final word could usefully be left to McGilloway and Donnelly (1977):

> . . . the patient is usually asked, 'Would you like to see the priest?' He is not usually asked if he would like to see the doctor, social worker, physiotherapist or any other member of the health care team. This process admirably illustrates the nurse's definition of the situation of the patient, chaplain and other health care personnel in the total care complex. It is possibly, primarily, a recognition of the patient's measure of control of this aspect of care, and does not necessarily reflect the practitioner's attitude towards the value of the chaplaincy service. This consideration becomes significant, however, if a chaplain is not called to any particular situation. It becomes particularly significant whenever the patient who has obvious needs, is required to request spiritual support, and whenever the patient whose needs are less obvious is required repeatedly to ask for spiritual help. It is not only that the patient may have a need to be helped in this way, but that the appropriate general pattern of action in regard to the source of help, is directly related to evaluation by nursing and other health care personnel who are inexpert in this field of care — of the general requirements of any patient situation. This evaluation may have important consequences regarding the completeness of patient care.

References

Balint, M (1957) The Doctor, His Patient and the Illness, Pitman Medical

Bowker, J (1970) Problems of Suffering in the Religions of the World, Cambridge University Press

Edwards, R B (1972) Reason and Religion — An Introduction to the Philosophy of Religion, Harcourt & Brace Jovanovich

Gabo, N (1959) Of Divers Arts, Faber & Faber

Hicks, J (1963) Philosophy of Religion, Prentice Hall

Isherwood, M (1970) Searching for Meaning — A Book for Agnostics and Believers, George Allen & Unwin

McGilloway, F A and Donnelly, L (1977) Religion and patient care — the functionalist approach, Journal of Advanced Nursing, 2: 3-13

Nigosian, S A (1975) World Religions, Edward Arnold

Stockwell, F (1970) The Unpopular Patient, Royal College of Nursing

Tillich, P (1951) Systematic Theology, Chicago University Press

Wilson M (1971) The Hospital, A Place of Truth — A Study of the Role of the Hospital Chaplain, University of Birmingham Institute for the Study of Worship and Religious Architecture

CHAPTER 10

NURSING MANAGEMENT OF LEISURE AND EMPLOYMENT

Following an investigation of stress factors in hospitals, Menzies (1970) claims that many hospitals contain large numbers of patients whose physical condition alone does not warrant hospitalization. 'In some cases', she writes, 'it is clear that these patients have been hospitalized because they and their relatives could not tolerate the stress of their being at home.' Such stress factors cannot centre solely on the patient's ability to carry out activities of daily living. The parameters of stress for the stroke victim and his family incorporate all aspects of living, including leisure and employment. Consequently, his progress in this area becomes a part of his overall assessment.

Concepts of leisure and free time

The term leisure is derived from the old French word *leisir*. It is usually defined as the time left over from work; however, in reality such time is only nominally free for leisure because of the time spent on self-maintenance and domestic duties.

Leisure may serve many purposes. Dumazdier (1967) indicates that it not only serves the purposes of rest, recreation and entertainment, but also the purpose of self-fulfilment. However, the planning schemes and architectural projects of local government tend not to focus on the self-fulfilment aspect of leisure; rather they emphasize more passive characteristics (Haworth 1975). Leisure is important for self-fulfilment because, as Roberts (1970) points out, the activities in which people participate during their free time play a significant part in the development of their sense of identity. He claims that it is only in their leisure lives that individuals feel they can express their real personality. Roberts believes that leisure-based attitudes and values are necessary to explain people's conduct in other spheres, and that, 'there are no sharp cleavages distinguishing the leisure activities of one situation of society from another'.

Burns (1973) claims that the way in which people spend their disposable money and time is a mode of organizing their lives, and that the concept of 'style of life' is more than a variable which is dependent upon social class or occupational status.

Cultural norms, inherited from the past, socialize us into a belief that work is good, and idleness reprehensible. This makes adjustment to sudden leisure difficult. The stroke victim, whether or not he is beyond the age of retirement, suddenly finds he appears to have gained in time usually free for leisure. However, free time and leisure are not one and the same thing. DeGrazia (1962) claims that free time refers to a special way of calculating time, but leisure refers to a state of being, a condition of man, which few desire and few achieve. Consequently, free time and leisure should not be measured by the same criteria. A stroke victim may have free time, but that is not synonymous with leisure.

The nurse, therefore, must examine what the concepts of free time and leisure mean for individual patients, because they will not mean the same to all people. Certain leisure activities are attractive to particular groups, not so much because of their intrinsic rewards, as for the social meaning which those activities have for those groups. We are influenced by our reference groups; we do the kind of things in our leisure time which 'our kind of people' do. We erect social filters around working men's clubs, golf clubs, discos and yacht clubs, to attract certain groups in and keep others out. This serves to give each person a unique mental leisure map of what is acceptable, and where he is acceptable and where not.

Having more free time does not necessarily lead to an automatic broadening of leisure activities. As people grow into middle age, their domestic responsibilities become lighter. Household chores become less demanding, and more money is usually available for leisure. During this phase of life, leisure interests might be expected to be rejuvenated, and people engage in more activities outside the home. For the wife in particular, release from the obligations of parental responsibility provides an increase in the amount of free time. However, Parker (1976) claims that very little increase in participative leisure takes place. Some people do develop an active interest in community-based organizations, such as church or civic associations, during their middle years, but Parker claims that this is not typical. The general trend is for leisure interests and activities to become increasingly restricted with age, despite decreased responsibilities.

Roberts (1970) offers two explanations for this decline in leisure activities. One is that during middle age the individual's physical and mental vigour declines, which may account for a reluctance to cultivate new interests. The second possible explanation, which Roberts offers, is that so many leisure industries aim to capture the interest of younger age groups; an image with which older people are reluctant to identify.

Single, middle-aged men and women can usually afford more expensive holidays and outings than a married couple on the same income. But many single people suffer from loneliness in their leisure hours. Just getting away on holiday is not always a solution for them, because they will be taking their loneliness with them on solitary holidays. They may prefer to immerse themselves in voluntary work, rather than face the emptiness of 'play' leisure.

Health and mobility have an important effect in both the amount of leisure available to an elderly person, and the quality of its enjoyment. Satisfying use of leisure, however, will not compensate for poor health, lost family or friends, or inadequate income (Brightbill 1960). Nor can it take the place of feelings of use-fulness and purposefulness, which are probably among the greatest needs of the stroke victim. The problem of filling time is partly solved for the stroke victim, in that simple activities take longer to do anyway. A nurse who intervenes and does things for the patient, rather than encouraging him to do things for himself, may be condemning him to many empty and meaningless hours.

The picture which emerged from a study by Smith (1971) was that the physically disabled have an above-average amount of disposable time, but are frustrated physically, mentally, environmentally and financially in their ability to enjoy this extra free time.

Monotony is an important and enduring human problem. Indeed, human beings are inclined actively to avoid a completely monotonous environment (Heron 1957). As people rest in isolation, cut off from stimulation, the content of their thoughts will gradually change. Heron claims that, in the first instance, an individual will consider present events and problems. After a while, he will begin to reminisce about past events, his family and friends. Eventually, lack of stimulation can lead to a state where concentration becomes too much of an effort, and the mind begins to drift, and blank periods intervene during which, the patient relates, he is not thinking of anything at all. Eagerness for stimulation may lead to the patient talking or singing to himself, and he may gradually become increasingly disorientated. Not only a lack of stimulation, but also a monotony of stimulation, can cause the emergence of this mental state. Monotonous repetition of any type, or amount of stimulation, will gradually lose the power of arousal. Simply switching on the radio or television will not overcome the monotony of a typical long-stay patient's day. A changing sensory environment is essential for all human beings, but it is particularly necessary for patients with long-term disabilities. Without it the brain ceases to function in an adequate and desirable way, and abnormalities of behaviour, such as childish emotional outbursts, may develop.

Any assessment of the leisure and recreational activities of the patient should take place within the context of the family as a whole. After all, family members, including husbands and wives, don't always get on well together. The impact of stroke on the lives of one couple is clearly illustrated by the following story, told to me by a social worker.

A professional man in his mid-fifties suffered a stroke, which left him with a hemiplegia and some speech disturbance. He and his wife had been prominent in the social circles of their community. The man appeared to be adjusting well to his disability, and seemed keen to become socially active again, in a limited way. However, the world of his wife had revolved around that of her husband. She had no social contacts of her own, and she was the one who could not adjust to the new style of life imposed by her husband's disability. She attempted to deny it existed, and would not take him out in a wheelchair, and hid any outward signs of disablement, such as ramps, from the view of the neighbours. Unable to resolve these conflicts, she resorted to drinking, and died of alcoholism a few years later.

Promoting social activity

The role of the rehabilitation centre

A modern rehabilitation centre is a busy and purposeful place. While no one pretends that a stroke victim can be 'cured', there is a likely expectation that life can continue to have meaning for the patient, especially if his mental capacity remains good. The staff of such centres are specially trained to give the patient plenty of time to attempt to do things for himself, and in making such attempts with minimal assistance. These centres give active treatment by way of medical care and nursing supervision; occupational, speech and physiotherapy; hydrotherapy, exercises and similar activities geared to increasing mobility. Patients can usually be resident or non-resident at such centres, and there is normally no time limit to their stay. Many rehabilitation centres have an assessment flat available, which totally simulates a home environment. The patient, and sometimes a close relative, live in this flat, under the indirect supervision of centre staff, for a number of days prior to discharge.

As has been pointed out earlier in this book, rehabilitation centres remain few in number, and are often long distances from the victim's domicile, which necessitates lengthy journeys by ambulance or other transport each day. Those who are resident at such centres will not have the support of family and friends but, conversely, in some instances the stroke victim may benefit from being away from an over-protective family. Unfortunately, admission to such centres is usually restricted, through referral by medical practitioners, to those who are continent and who have a good prognosis. Even a suitable stroke victim may not receive the restorative facilities of such a centre if the doctor is not aware of the availability of these facilities or does not support a philosophy of rehabilitation. There is no evidence that such a philosophy pervades the medical and nursing profession.

Any climate richer and less sterile than the medical environment can be useful for a variety of therapeutic group activities. It would seem that psychological adjustments, sharing of feelings, learning new skills, and generally giving support to one another, demands a climate which is freer and less tense, for stroke victims, than can be found in acute medical wards.

The stroke team

The value of a specialist stroke team, outside a rehabilitation centre, has been recognized by several authors. Brocklehurst et al. (1981), for example, claim that there is a case for the development of such teams, to form a mobile force which could be called out, at short notice, to give advice and practical help to stroke victims and their families. The objectives of a stroke team should be as follows:

1   To identify facilities, especially community resources, for use in recovery in stroke.

2   To teach the concepts and advantages of rehabilitation to health service personnel.

3   To demonstrate the feasibility of using surrogates, including volunteers, when specialized rehabilitation personnel are not available.

4   To support the efforts of staff and relatives to continue to deliver rehabilitative services to stroke victims, in the absence of the stroke team.

While there is a consensus among authors as to the value of a stroke team, there are differences of opinion as to who should lead the team, and its composition. It is the opinion of this author that the stroke team should be based upon a core of hospital and community nurses, who are trained in rehabilitative techniques to the level of clinical specialist. They could be coordinated by a nurse administrator. For each patient, especially if he is not able to be his own advocate, a family coordinator should be included (Figure 10.1).

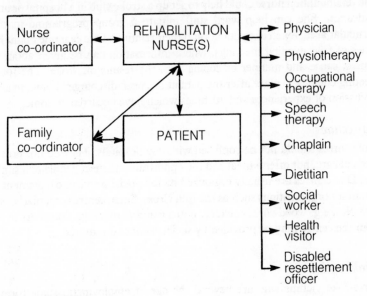

Figure 10.1 The stroke team

The nurse should be responsible for procedures to prevent contractures, maintain mobility, prevent pressure sores and promote continence, good personal hygiene and nutrition. She should also be responsible for promoting social opportunities for the patient. The nurse would consult with the other members of the team, and call upon their specialized knowledge, when appropriate to the needs of the individual patient.

There may be early problems in getting a stroke team to function as a unit, but these can be overcome by cooperative effort and confident personal relationships. The members of the stroke team should be chosen because of their commitment to the concept of rehabilitation, and because of their interpersonal skills, which will be necessary to circumvent any obstructive forces within the health services. The rehabilitation nurse must have the ability to work through the many internal problems with administrative, medical and nursing personnel, before she can function effectively as a teacher, principal deliverer of care, as a careful observer, and as an evangelist on behalf of restorative care (Kahn 1971).

The stroke team should be available to advise hospital staff in the care of their stroke patients, and respond quickly to calls for help in the community. The rehabilitation nurse could help to set up a stroke club in a hospital or other institution. She can help ward staff initiate a group programme in their particular area, for stroke patients and their relatives. One example might be a series of four evening meetings, where information can be given about the nature, cause and manner of coping with the results of stroke. The fourth meeting could take place after the patient has been discharged home, to allow discussion of experiences and attitudes which have occurred at home.

Day centres

Day centres should not be confused with day hospitals. They do not provide medical care, but offer a meal and the opportunity to meet people of a similar age. Day centres are usually organized by the Social Services department, or voluntary organizations such as the Red Cross. Some centres organize special activities, e.g. woodwork, cookery, pottery and gardening. Transport to and from the centre may be provided by social services if required.

Stroke clubs

For stroke victims who are beyond the age of employment, some form of continuing rehabilitation is necessary to prevent regression and possible commitment to long-term care. To this end, several hundred Stroke Clubs have been set up countrywide, by volunteer workers, often with the advice of the Chest, Heart and Stroke Association, which maintains an up-to-date list of such centres. Stroke Clubs offer socio-educational opportunities for both stroke victims and their relatives. The majority of clubs meet once a month in a local church or community hall. This social outlet can act as an important safety valve for the carer. McCormick and Williams (1975) claim that, 'the chronic effects of stroke appear virtually to destroy the life style of families, more often than should be tolerated'.

Wives in particular often feel that no one seems to really understand how difficult it is for them to change their lifestyles to care for their husbands. Many health professionals tend to take it for granted that a housewife would have few problems in adapting to the needs of her partner. However, the housewife may be called upon to serve the multiple roles of psychologist, social worker, pharmacist, physiotherapist, nurse, speech therapist, lover, domestic, social secretary or dietitian. These women may be existing on the thin edge of sanity. Safilios-Rothschild (1970) claims that married women who become disabled, especially those with children, are usually taken back into the family, and even if severely impaired, tend to maintain a part of their usual role function. Supportive services, and the assistance of neighbours and friends, appear more readily forthcoming to help the husband as opposed to the wife of a stroke victim. One possible explanation for this extra eagerness to provide assistance for the husband may be the stereotype of domestic helplessness of the male. Perhaps this is why more wives desert their disabled husbands, than husbands abandon their disabled wives. The wife is especially likely to leave home if she has a desire to perform a social or vocational role.

The single disabled person tends to be more independent in daily living activities, than married disabled individuals, usually because of necessity. Nevertheless, they may need the social outlet of a Stroke Club even more than a married couple.

The Stroke Club provides a form of group therapy and group support. Club members are encouraged to take part in group games such as beetle drives. Non-verbal games such as noughts and crosses, draughts and dominoes, can allow a receptive aphasic patient to play as an equal, especially if he played such games before his stroke. Local Social Service departments may agree to provide transport to the club; otherwise the organizers maintain a list of voluntary drivers.

Stroke Clubs can also be formed in hospitals, especially those hospitals concerned with long-term care. Hoff (1971) claims that all patients are more likely to be more stimulated, and participate more actively, in the company of outsiders, than with the same people whom they see every day. Nurses and therapists can arrange a variety of group activities in a convenient room of the hospital. All stroke victims should be invited to attend if there is no clinical contradiction to prevent their involvement. Whenever possible, some of the activitives should take place at a time when relatives can join in. I recall an instance where a games activity on a ward stopped at visiting hour. A stroke victim who had been taking part with obvious enjoyment was then wheeled to meet a visiting relative. The two sat in almost total silence for about 30 minutes, before the visitor made some excuse and left. Both could perhaps have enjoyed the visit more if they had been encouraged to do something together, or share the activities of staff and other patients.

Each session should not last more than 2 hours because of the risk of fatigue. Whenever possible the patients should initiate activities. The occupational therapist could assist the patients in making a variety of games suitable for hemiplegic players. For example, a simple dart board with rubber tipped darts, or a set of nine pin bowls and soft balls with which to knock them down. One bean bag game, which is usually popular and inexpensive, consists of a number of old tins of different diameters, which are numbered, with the largest tin being designated the lowest score. The tins are placed on the floor in the centre of a circle of stroke patients, and if the patient can throw the bean bag into a tin, he adds the number on that tin to his score. Such games may appear somewhat childish to the able bodied, but they help to improve the patient's hand and eye coordination, and simply getting the bag into a tin may represent an enormous achievement to a severe stroke victim.

As well as games, physiotherapy exercises might be conducted to rhythmical music, in follow-my-leader style. Staff and relatives can join in the fun. Some patients may find expression in painting or drawing. The birthdays of club members could be celebrated in some special way. Eventually, a spirit of cohesion and belonging should materialize. Sharing group activities can act as a stimulus to both sexes. This will become apparent through more careful grooming, sustained attendance at the club, and examples of solicitude for the comfort and welfare of others. Initially, long-stay female patients may need encouraging before they will take part because, as Gordon and Vinacke (1971) claim, women appear to accept dependency more readily than males.

Gardening

Gardening is important for its therapeutic value, and is an enjoyable hobby for a stroke victim. However, there is a tendency for disabled males to give up this activity following stroke.

If circumstances allow, a small garden might be set up between two wards, or a number of growing boxes could be arranged in a courtyard. A small potting shed, arranged so that everything comes easily to hand, might be erected by volunteers. If space allows, a greenhouse, large enough for ease of access, can provide an alternative opportunity for gardening, or a winter pastime.

Volunteer groups, such as the British Voluntary Service, may be able to help the stroke victim with his garden at home. Such help will often encourage the patient to take an active interest in his garden, whereas if left to his own resources he may lose heart.

The main aim should be simplicity, and keeping the number of laborious tasks to a minimum. By substituting permanent year round plants with those demanding seasonal planting, interest and involvement can be sustained all year round. Digging can be made easier with a Terrex spade, which requires no bending or lifting. Soil levels can be raised and retained by edging with stones or logs. Stone troughs, tubs or large flower pots can be raised up on bricks. Compost making can be changed from traditional methods, to one using a compost bin, which produces liquified manure. Before the stroke victim begins gardening, all paths and steps should be inspected to ensure that uneven surfaces will not cause accidents.

Driving a car

Whether or not a stroke victim is able to drive again will depend on the type of stroke he has had, and the severity of his residual disability. If his disability lasts more than 3 months, he is legally obliged to inform the Driving Licensing Authority, on a special form obtainable from the Post Office. He may have to take a special driving test before he can resume driving. Patients with obvious hemiplegia, hemianopia or transient ischaemic attacks, should never be allowed to drive any motorized vehicle.

Employment

Vocational rehabilitation is a much longer process than medical rehabilitation. Smolkin and Cohen (1974) reveal that lack of education plays a significant role in inhibiting vocational rehabilitation among stroke victims. They claim that women in particular tend to have less potential for vocational rehabilitation among the less educated groups. Prior occupation appears to exert a major influence on a successful return to work, especially within the professional, technical and managerial areas. Weisbroth et al. (1971) claim that one third of stroke victims in their study returned to some form of competitive employment. They found that there was no significant difference between left and right hemiplegia in this respect. However, the least successful group were patients suffering left hemiplegia with impaired articulation and decreased abstract reasoning.

The responsibility for finding employment for young stroke victims rests mainly with the Disabled Resettlement Officer (DRO). Assessment for employment should begin early. Psychological testing is not advocated because, as Lyman (1963) points out, such tests are of limited value in predicting the outcome of vocational success. Rather than psychological or another form of testing, the patient should be asked to attempt samples of work in the occupational therapy department. Such samples might include actual work taken from the office, factory or other facility. Eventually, the patient might be placed in an actual work situation, e.g. clerical work, cashier, carpentry, electronics or assembly work.

The Disabled Resettlement Officer normally works from an employment or job centre. He is a part of the staff of the Training Services Agency, of the Manpower Services Commission. His role is to interview disabled persons, including stroke victims, and if possible find them suitable work within their previous employment, or an alternative placement in a special vacancy reserved for disabled persons. He may recommend some form of retraining. The DRO is an invaluable ally because he understands disablement, and its medical, social and economic consequences. Once he has found employment for the person, he monitors the progress of the individual in the working environment.

Smolkin and Cohen (1974) claim that for the moderately to severely disabled stroke population, a team effort of rehabilitation specialists might have advantage over routine handling, especially in terms of vocational outcome.

References

Brightbill, CK (1960) The Challenge of Leisure, Prentice Hall

Brocklehurst, J C, Morris, P, Andrews, K, Richards, B and Laycock, P (1981) Social effects of stroke, Social Science and Medicine, 15A: 35-39.

Burns, T (1973) Leisure in industrial society, in M A Smith, S R Parker and C S Smith (Editors) Leisure in Britain, Allen Lane

DeGrazia, S (1962) Of Time, Work and Leisure, Twentieth Century Fund

Dumazedier, J (1967) Towards a Society of Leisure, The Free Press

Gordon, S K and Vinacke, W E (1971) Self and ideal concepts and dependency in aged persons residing in institutions, Journal of Gerontology, 26 (3): 337-343

Haworth, J J (1975) Human needs, work and leisure, in J J Haworth and M A Smith (Editors) Work and Leisure, Lepus Books

Heron, W (1957) The pathology of boredom, Scientific American, 196 (1): 52-56

Hoff, A A (1971) A post stroke success story in the rehabilitation of hospitalised elderly patients, Medical Annals of the District of Columbia, 40 (10): 640-643

Kahn, R R (1971) Stroke rehabilitation in general hospitals, Hospitals (Chicago), 45: 47-49

Lyman, H B (1963) Test Scores and What They Mean, Prentice Hall

McCormick, G P and Williams, M (1975) Stroke — the double crisis, American Journal of Nursing, 75 (8): 1410-1411

Menzies, I E P (1970) The Functioning of Social Systems as a Defence Against Anxiety, Tavistock Institute for Human Relations, London

Parker, S (1976) The Sociology of Leisure, George Allen & Unwin

Roberts, K (1970) Leisure, Longman

Safilios-Rothschild, C (1970) The Sociology and Social Psychology of Disability and Rehabilitation, Random House

Smith, C R W (1971) Leisure activities in impaired persons, in A Harris et al. (Editor) Handicapped and Impaired in Great Britain, HMSO

Smolkin, C and Cohen, B S (1974) Socio- economic factors affecting the vocational success of stroke patients, Archives of Physical Medicine and Rehabilitation, 55: 269-271

Weisbroth, S, Esibill, N and Zuger, R R (1971) Factors in vocational success of hemiplegic patients, Archives of Physical Medicine and Rehabilitation, 52: 441-446

CHAPTER 11

NURSING MANAGEMENT OF SEXUALITY

Sexuality and ageing

In a review of the nursing literature on human sexuality, Brower and Tanner (1979) claim that most nursing authors are not concerned over nursing implications of sexuality, particularly in older individuals. As nursing embraces a holistic concept of care, the sexual dimension of the older patient deserves more consideration. Many stroke victims are elderly, therefore several general considerations can apply equally to them. Problems of sexuality are also prominent among young stroke victims, who tend to be males, and who may have many years of disability ahead of them.

Nurses as members of a predominantly 'young' profession are for the most part recruited from, and working in, a youth-orientated society. Such a society emphasizes attractiveness, vigour and productivity, and nowhere is this more apparent than in the area of human sexuality (Spennrath 1982). Many people, both old and young, express astonishment at the concept of human beings in their 70s, 80s or even 90s making love. Youth is generally disdainful of sexual interest in the elderly and, consequently, there is no group in society more widely discriminated against in terms of their sexuality than the old.

Culturally derived stereotypes, fostered by negative attitudes towards ageing, have been responsible for the abundance of myths, contributing to a prevailing resistance to acceptance of sexuality in the elderly. An example of such a myth would be that sexual desire ceases with the menopause. Consequently, for some individuals, the myth of the sexless years after 65 becomes a self-fulfilling prophecy. Other elderly people who continue to experience a strong sex drive may feel guilt and shame, because they believe such a state is abnormal. What is labelled virility at 25 becomes lechery at 65 (Burnside 1973). Masturbation, which may have been practised as a means of relieving sexual tension for decades, suddenly becomes 'infantile' behaviour.

Many such myths have become formalized into institutional practices, which in turn reinforce a stereotyped approach towards sexual matters. Shomaker (1980), for example, claims that doctors and nurses are unwilling to take sexual histories of people over 60 years of age, especially single women, because they feel that sex does not exist for these persons. In long-stay hospitals or residential homes, contact between single persons of both sexes is often restricted to public areas where the behaviour of the residents can be observed. Any overt display of sexual behaviour is usually frowned upon and may lead to further segregation.

A need for close, intimate contact with another human being is present from birth, and never diminishes in intensity or meaningfulness. Throughout the life cycle, each person needs another human being to respond to him, whether by intellectual exchanges, or by engagement of the body, as in touching, patting, stroking, hugging and, sometimes, sexual intercourse (Diekelmann 1977). However, research has suggested that among the different age groups, it is the elderly who receive the least amount of touching from health personnel (Hollinger 1980).

The majority of older adults have some concern about sex. In the case of men, this is often associated with fear of loss of potency (Spennrath 1982). For women, such concern centres on the loss of physical attractiveness to the opposite sex, exemplified by the expansion of industries concerned with supporting stereotypes of beauty, such as cosmetic surgery.

Although there is a gradual decline in the reproductive capability of women after the age of 30, there is no physiological change that rings down a mandatory curtain on sexuality in either men or women. In males over 60, there is a general reduction in the level of the hormone testosterone circulating in the body. In addition, spermatogenesis will begin to diminish after 50, but continues into the ninth decade. Men over 60 usually require more direct genital stimulation to achieve and maintain a firm erection. It may take longer for the man to complete the sex act, and the intensity of the orgasm may be somewhat decreased. Men between the ages of 60 and 90 may find sexual intercourse without ejaculation satisfying (Horbert and Ginsberg 1979).

Interest in sex among women may increase rather than decrease after the menopause, because of a lack of concern about pregnancy. However 75% of women over 65 are no longer sexually active, compared with 25% of males. Reasons cited for male inactivity include impotence, sickness and lack of interest. Women tend to be sexually inactive because they have no partners. The death of the husband, or his illness, divorce or separation, or lack of interest, are the most frequently cited reasons why this should be so. Therefore, while there is no biological limitation to the sexual capacity in the female, the majority of women over 65 have to terminate or adapt their sex lives, not because of personal preference, or individual disability, but as a direct or indirect consequence of the structures and norms of society. This does not appear to be the situation for the male. The average woman can expect to live about 25 years after the menopause, and she is more likely to outlive her partner, yet there appears to be no socially sanctioned form of normal sexual activity available to her. As Diekelmann (1977) points out:

> It is little wonder that old women, frequently deprived of their males, through having outlived them, separated from family members, both in terms of physical and emotional disturbance, as a result of our mobile population with its emphasis on nuclear families, separated from meaningful employment, by mandatory retirement, and experiencing increasing dependence because of chronic health problems, should have tremendous needs for some expression of affection and concern from another human being.

The efforts of the elderly to attain some semblance of physical closeness by touching should not be viewed as unhealthy or obscene, but as the expression of a normal human drive, and as a plea for recognition as a human being.

Following stroke, sexual activity may present a wide array of physical and psychological difficulties for both partners. A few male victims may be physically incapable of intercourse, but they may well be able to resume an active sex life by other means. The male stroke victim will be concerned that his masculinity is at risk. He will worry that he might become impotent, that he will not be able to achieve or maintain an erection. The female victim will worry that her hemiplegia or communication problems will render her unattractive to her partner, or other males. A distorted body image may compound such fears.. The wife of a stroke victim is often afraid to respond to the advances of her husband, out of concern for his health. She may worry that sexual intercourse may precipitate another stroke, and her husband may interpret this as a lack of interest, putting at risk his concept of himself as a man. It may be up to the partner of the stroke victim to make the first move to demonstrate affection.

If the patient is hypertensive he may be receiving medication. Several common hypotensive drugs have side effects which cause inhibition or delay in ejaculation.

Counselling

Staff and family members often become upset when *their* expectations of the sexual behaviour of elderly or disabled persons are not met. Before a nurse assumes the role of counsellor, she must have her own attitudes and feelings under control. Unfortunately, the opportunities to explore such attitudes to human sexuality in nurse education programmes remain few. If the nurse attempts counselling from a platform of her own stereotyped images of sexuality in the elderly, there is a high risk that she may impose her own values on the patient. Differences in age, or a lack of necessary knowledge, may make it difficult for a nurse to manipulate the subject in an effective way, to meet the needs of an individual, or married couple.

Counselling should begin with the client's level of readiness, and not that of the nurse. When the suitability of the moment becomes apparent, the nurse should arrange a warm and accepting atmosphere, in an environment where privacy and freedom from intrusion is assured. Any assessment of the sexual needs of the patient should take place against a background of knowledge of his life situation. The objective of counselling is to help the patient, and his partner, to find a satisfactory outlet for sexual desires, not necessarily through sexual intercourse. Sex by itself cannot be a substitute for intimacy. Sexual needs can be met by alternative measures, such as touching, kissing, embracing, fantasizing or masturbation. Simply having the opportunity to enjoy the company of the opposite sex may be sufficient.

If the husband has hemiplegia, he may not be able to support himself in the usual position to achieve intercourse. The couple may be advised to adopt an alternative position to overcome this problem, such as the man lying on his side, or the woman assuming the upper position. The use of sexual aids might be discussed with the couple. Vibrators, for example, can be useful to increase stimulation. The energy expended in the sex act is equivalent to climbing two flights of stairs or going for a brisk walk, so there should be little likelihood that sexual intercourse will precipitate a second stroke in the husband. However, the man should not attempt intercourse if he feels tired, after a heavy meal, or if he has been drinking alcohol.

Unless the patient has had a severe stroke, which demands prolonged nursing intervention, the couple should be encouraged to retain their double bed for as long as possible.

In situations where sexual intercourse is not possible, or desirable, the nurse should consider how she might manipulate the environment to allow individuals to express their sexuality, through arranging activities in which both sexes can take part.

References

Brower, H T and Tanner, L A (1979) A study of older adults attending a programme on human sexuality — a pilot study, Nursing Research, 28(1): 36-39

Burnside, I M (1973) Sexuality and ageing, Medical Arts and Sciences, 27 (3): 13-27

Diekelmann, N (1977) Primary Health Care of the Well Adult, McGraw-Hill

Hollinger, L M (1980) Perception of touch in the elderly, Journal of Gerontological Nursing, 6: 741-746

Horbert, A S and Ginsberg, L H (1979) Human Services for Older Adults — Concepts and Skills, Wadsworth

Shomaker, D M (1980) Integration of physiological and sociocultural factors as a basis for sex education in the elderly, Journal of Gerontological Nursing, 6: 311-318

Spennrath, S (1982) Understanding the sexual needs of the older patient, Canadian Nurse, 78 (7): 25-29

GLOSSARY

Acalculia (also **Dyscalculia**) A disturbance in the use of mathematical symbols

ADL Activities of daily living

Ageusia Impairment of taste

Agnosia Failure to recognize familiar objects perceived by the senses

Agrammatism A reduction in the ability to form intelligible sentences

Agraphia (also **Dysgraphia**) Inability to express oneself in writing

Ahylognosia Inability to differentiate qualities of materials

Akinetic mutism Unresponsiveness to the environment

Alexia (also **Dyslexia**) A difficulty in reading, sometimes called 'word blindness'

Amaurosis fugax Transient monocular blindness

Amusia A defect in auditory perception involving loss of musical appreciation

Anarthria (see **Dysarthria**)

Anomia Inability to name familiar objects and family names

Anosmia Loss of ability to identify odours

Anosodiaphoria Patient shows no concern about his paralysis

Anosognosia A severe form of neglect in which the patient fails to recognize or denies his paralysis (not caused by loss of memory)

Anton's Syndrome Visual denial

Aphasia (also **Dysphasia**) Inability to express oneself through speech, or the inability to comprehend the spoken word

Types of aphasia include:

Amnesic Nominal
Anomic Loss of ability to name familiar objects
Auditory Word deafness
Expressive (also *Broca's*) Lack of verbal expression
Central Syntactical
Fluent Receptive
Global Loss of all communication functions
Graphomotor Inability to write
Lichteim's Loss of spontaneous speech, but not ability to repeat words
Nominal Loss of ability to name objects
Non-fluent Expressive
Receptive (also *Wernicke's*) Loss of ability to comprehend verbal or written symbols
Semantic Inability to recognize the significance of words
Syntactical Inability to speak sequentially
Tactile Inability to name objects touched
Transcortical Ability to repeat words

Apraxia Inability to perform certain purposeful movements, e.g. dressing, without loss of motor power, sensation or coordination.
Types of apraxia include:

Constructional Inability to copy simple designs
Ideational Inability to carry out a complex act
Ideomotor The patient has some knowledge of how to do it, but not correctly
Kinetic Instinctive grasping

Astereognosis Loss of ability to recognize objects when handling with eyes closed
Asymbolia Inability to comprehend and use words, gestures, and/or any type of symbols
Asynergia Lack of coordination of muscles in voluntary actions
Ataxia Lack of coordination in voluntary motion
Autopagnosia Loss of ability to locate a sensation through lack of recognition of body parts
Bobath method An attempt to change abnormal patterns of posture and movement by using 'key points' of control

Body image   The patient's mental representation of his body, expressing his feelings and thoughts about his body, rather than representing an exact picture of the physical structure

Body scheme   A postural model of himself; how he perceives the position of the body, and the relationship of body parts

Broca's aphasia   See **Aphasia**

Brunnstrom method   An attempt to improve function through positioning and pathologic reflexes

Cerebral embolism   A sudden plugging of a cerebral blood vessel by a clot

Cerebral haemorrhage   Bleeding into the tissue of the brain

Cerebral thrombosis   Formation or presence of intravascular material in a cerebral artery, obstructing the blood flow

Clonus   Interrupted muscle contraction caused by alternating rigidity and relaxation in rapid succession

Completed stroke   A stroke in which clinical signs and symptoms have become stable

Confabulation   Readily answers to questions without regard for truthfulness

Confusion   Mingling of ideas, with a loss of understanding

CVA   Cerebral vascular accident; a sudden diminution of the blood supply to the brain

Dementia   Mental and intellectual deterioration

Diploplia   Double vision; perception of two images of an object

Disability   Reduction in function as a result of impairment

Dysarthria   (also **Anarthria**) Inability to control the movement or coordination of organs of speech; slurring of consonants; variation of stress and speed of speech

Dyscalculia   see **Acalculia**

Dysgraphia   see **Agraphia**

Dyslexia   see **Alexia**

Dysphagia   Difficulty in swallowing

Dysphasia   see **Aphasia**

Dyspraxia   see **Apraxia**

Expressive aphasia   see **Aphasia**

Echolalia   Transcortical receptive aphasia; meaningless repetition by patients, of words addressed to him

Gerstmann's syndrome   A syndrome believed to be derived from a lesion in the dominant hemisphere involving difficulty in writing and calculation, lack of discrimination between right and left, and doubt and hesitation concerning the use of fingers

Hemianaesthesia Disturbance of all sensations in trunk and limbs on one side of the body

Hemianopia ((also **Hemianopsia**) Defective vision of half of the visual field
Homonymous hemianopia Both right halves or both left halves of the visual field are affected

Hemiparesis Muscular weakness on one side of the body

Hemiplegia Paralysis on one side of the body

Impairment Variation from normal anatomy or function

Ingravescent stroke A 'stroke-in-evolution'; a stroke in which the symptoms are progressing

Lacunae A softening of the tissue surrounding damaged cerebral vessels, found at autopsy in many hemiplegics

Limbic system The part of the brain that maintains behaviour patterns; includes the olfactory bulb, mamillary body, fornix and hippocampus

Macrosomatognosia A disorder in body scheme that distorts the patient's perception of his body, making him see it as abnormally large

Metamorphia A distortion in the size and shape of objects; usually found in lesions of the parietal lobe

Paragraphia Mistakes in spelling or the use of the wrong words in writing

Paralexia The inappropriate transposition of words or syllables in reading

Parosomia Interference with smell

Perception The ability to interpret sensory messages from the internal and external environment, so that the sensation has meaning

Perseveration The continuation of an activity or movement after its stimulus has been removed

Position sense Ability to identify the position of a limb in space with eyes closed

Prosopagnosia Inability to recognize differences in faces

Receptive aphasia see **Aphasia**

Reflex An involuntary movement resulting from an afferent impulse
Types of reflex include the following:

Babinski Dorsiflexion of the big toe following stimulation of the sole of the foot

Bulbomimic Pressure on the eyeball of a comatose hemiplegic causes contraction of the facial muscles on the opposite side to the lesion

Brain An extension of the hemiplegic flexed arm when the patient tries to get onto all fours

Magnus and de Kleijn An increase in upper limb tonus on the side to which the chin is turned

Myotatic Stretch reflex

Palmomental The corner of the mouth twitches when the palm on the same side is pricked with a pin.

Righting A return to a balanced position if balance is suddenly disturbed

Stretch A contraction of muscle following longitudinal stretch

Tonic A muscle contraction which persists for some time after stimulus is removed

Shoulder-hand syndrome Pain, stiffness, swelling and disturbance of upper limb; probably an autonomic nervous system disturbance

Simultanagnosia Spatial disorientation; perseveration; and amnesia

Somatognosia Unawareness of body structure, and failure to recognize body parts and their relationships to each other

Spasticity An increase in muscle tone with exaggerated tendon reflexes and increased reponse to passive stretch

Stroke An acute deprivation of the supply of blood to part of the brain

Speech processes Includes five motor elements: respiration, phonation, articulation, resonance and prosody

Subarachnoid haemorrhage A bleeding into the subarachnoid space, usually as a result of a burst aneurysm at the base of the brain

Subclavian steel A reversal of the blood flow in a vertebral artery

Synkinesis Unilateral movement of one limb when motion is willed in the other; usually symmetrical

TIA Transient ischaemic attack; a short lasting, reversible set of symptoms resulting from interference with cerebral blood supply

Wernicke's aphasia see **Aphasia**

BIBLIOGRAPHY

Pathophysiology

Benson, B F and Tomlinson, E B (1971) Hemiplegic syndrome of the posterior cerebral artery, Stroke, 2: 559

Heilman, M (1974) Neurophysiologic changes in the stroke patient, Geriatrics, 29, Feb: 153-160

McCormick, W F and Rosenfeld, D B (1973) Massive brain haemorrhage — a review of 144 cases and examination of their causes, Stroke, 4: 876

Marshall, J (1974) Types of hemiplegia, Physiotherapy, 60 (11): 334-335

Wallhagen, M I (1979) The split brain — implications for care and rehabilitation, American Journal of Nursing, 79 (12): 2118-2125

Clinical deficits following stroke

Albert, M L (1973) A simple test for visual neglect, Neurology, 23: 658

Anderson, E K (1971) Sensory impairment in hemiplegia, Archives of Physical Medicine and Rehabilitation, 52: 293

Haerer, A F (1973) Visual field defects and prognosis of stroke patients, Stroke, 4: 163

Huston, J (1975) Overcoming learning disabilities of stroke, Nursing 75 (5) Sept: 66-68

Isaacs, B (1973) When a stroke patient draws a picture — a clue to disability, Geriatrics, 28: 101

Johnson, J H and Cryan, M (1979) Homonymous hemianopsia — assessment and management, American Journal of Nursing, 79 (12): 2131-2134

Lucas, M (1969) Perceptual disorders of adults with hemiplegia, Physical Therapy, 49: 1078-1083

Newman, M (1972) The process of recovery after stroke, Stroke, 3: 702

Piggott, R and Brickett, F (1966) Visual neglect, American Journal of Nursing, 66, Jan: 101

Rubin, R (1968) Body image and self esteem, Nursing Outlook, 16, June: 20-23

Siev, E and Friestadt, B (1976) Perceptual Dysfunction in the Adult Stroke Patient, Charles B Slack

Ullman, M (1964) Disorders of body image after stroke, American Journal of Nursing, 64, Oct: 98

Posture and mobility

Bramwell Jones, S (1969) The household needs of the disabled — a guide to the selection of furniture and equipment, British Hospital Journal Social Services Review, 79: 679

Browse, N S (1965) Physiology and Pathology of Bedrest, Charles C Thomas

Ellams, R (1973) After stroke — sitting problems, American Journal of Nursing, 73, Nov: 1898-1899

Feeney, R J and Galer, M (1978) Selecting aids for disabled people, National Corporation for the Care of Old People, London

Fenwick, D (1977) Wheelchairs and their users, Office of Populations, Censuses and Surveys, HMSO

Kern, F C and Pool, L (1972) Transfer techniques, Nursing, 72: 25

Lockhart, T (1982) Housing Adaptations for Disabled People, The Architectural Press

Snyder, M and Baum, R (1974) Assessing station and gait, American Journal of Nursing, 74, July: 1256-1257

Wells, K F (1966) Kinesiology, W B Saunders

Williams, N (1967) Correlation between copying ability and dressing activities in hemiplegia, American Journal of Physical Medicine, 46: 1332

Nutrition

Beck, M E (1975) Nutrition and Dietetics for Nurses, 4th edition, Churchill Livingstone

Bennion, M (1969) Clinical Nutrition, Harper & Row

Gaffrey, T W and Campbell, M (1974) Feeding techniques for dysphagic patients, American Journal of Nursing, 74: 2194-2195

Grant, M M and Kubo, W M (1975) Assessing a patient's hydration status, American Journal of Nursing, 75, Aug: 1306-1312

Howard, R B and Herbold, N H (eds) (1978) Nutrition in Clinical Care, McGraw-Hill

Howe, P S (1971) Basic Nutrition in Health and Disease — Including Selection and Care of Food, W B Saunders

Joint FAO/WHO Expert Group (1967) Requirements of Vitamin A, Thiamine, Riboflavine and Niacin, Food and Agricultural Organization of the United Nations

Porter, J W G and Rolls, B A (eds) (1973) Proteins in Human Nutrition, Academic Press

Royal College of Physicians (1980) Medical Aspects of Dietary Fibre, Pitman Medical

Webster, G D (1970) Foods and fluids for the stroke patient — current concepts of cerebral vascular disease, American Heart Association, 5: 25

Winick, M (1980) Nutrition in Health and Disease, J Wiley & Sons

Elimination

Adams, B, Baron, M and Caston, M A (1966) Urinary incontinence in the acute phase of cerebral vascular accident, Nursing Research, 15: 100

Habbeb, M and Kallstrom, M (1976) Bowel program for institutionalized adults, American Journal of Nursing, 76, April: 606

Tudor, L L (1970) Bladder and bowel retraining, American Journal of Nursing, 70: 2391

Whittington, L (1980) Bladder retraining, Canadian Nurse, 76 (6): 26-29

Willington, F L (1981) Cleansing incontinent patients — an evaluation of the use of non-ionic detergents compared with soap, Journal of Advanced Nursing, 6 (2): 107-111

Wright, L (1974) Bowel Function in Hospital Patients, Royal College of Nursing

Personal hygiene

Bliss, M and McLaren, R (1967) Preventing pressure sores in geriatric patients, Nursing Mirror, 123: 434-437

Bretton, P (1974) Aids for bathing the disabled, Nursing Times, 70: 1741-1745

Carney, R (1963) The ageing skin, American Journal of Nursing, 63: 110-112

Ewing, M R, Garrow, C and McHugh, N (1961) Sheepskin as a nursing aid, Lancet, 2: 1147

Simko, M (1967) Foot welfare, American Journal of Nursing, 67: 1895-1897

Tassman, G C, Zayon, G M and Zafron, J N (1963) When patients cannot brush their teeth, American Journal of Nursing, 63, Feb:76

Sleep and rest

Bassler, S (1974) The origins and development of biological rhythms, Nursing Clinics of North America, 11: 575-582

Downs, F S (1974) Bedrest and sensory disturbances, American Journal of Nursing, 74: 2316-2330

Fass, G (1971) Sleep, drugs and dreams, American Journal of Nursing, 71: 2310-2320

Freeman, F R (1974) Sleep Research — A Critical Review, 2nd edition, Charles C Thomas

Hartmann, E (1975) Sleep requirements — long sleepers, short sleepers, variable sleepers and insomniacs, Psychosomatics, 14: 95-103

Horne, J A and Porter, J M (1975) Exercise and human sleep, Nature, 256: 573-574

McGhie, A and Russell, S (1962) The subjective assessment of normal sleep patterns, Journal of Mental Science, 108: 642-654

Norris, C M (1975) Restlessness — a nursing phenomena in search of meaning, Nursing Outlook, 23, Feb: 103-107

Williams, R L, Karacan, I and Hursch, C J (1974) EEG and Human Sleep — Clinical Applications, J Wiley & Sons

Spiritual comfort

Cartwright, A (1964) Human Relations and Hospital Care, Routledge & Kegan Paul

Chapman, C M (1980) The rights and responsibilities of nurses and patients, Journal of Advanced Nursing, 5 (2): 127-134

Schrock, R A (1980) A question of honesty in nursing practice, Journal of Advanced Nursing, 5(2): 135-148

Stoll, R I (1979) Guidelines for spiritual behaviour, American Journal of Nursing, 79, Sept: 1574-1577

Weatherhead, L D (1951) Psychology, Religion and Healing, Hodder & Stoughton

Communication

Amacher, N I (1973) Touch is a way of caring — and a way of communicating with an aphasic patient, American Journal of Nursing, 73, Mar: 852

Barrett, K (1972) A survey of the current utilization of touch by health team personnel with hospitalized patients, International Journal of Nursing Studies, 9, Nov: 195

Cohen, L K (1971) Communication Problems After Stroke, Kenny Rehabilitation Centre, Minneapolis

Culton, G L (1969) Spontaneous recovery from aphasia, Journal of Speech and Hearing Research, 12: 825

Darley, F (1972) The efficiency of language rehabilitation in aphasia, Journal of Speech and Hearing Disorders, 37:3

Fox, M J (1976) Patients with receptive aphasia, American Journal of Nursing, 76, Oct: 1596-1598

Harrington, R (1975) Communication for the aphasic stroke patient — assessment and therapy, Journal of the American Geriatrics Society, 23 (6): 254-257

Kron, T (1972) How do we communicate non verbally with patients? Canadian Nurse, 68, Nov: 23

Mason, A and Pratt, J (1980) Touch, Nursing Times, 76 (23): 999-1001

Raemakers, Sister M J (1979) Communication blocks revisited, American Journal of Nursing, 79, June, 1079-1080

Sarno, M T and Hook, O (eds) (1980)Aphasia — Assessment and Treatment, Almqvist & Wiksell International

Wohl, M T (1969) Disorders of communication, Nursing Mirror, 128 (11): 20

Socializing

Falknor, H M and Harris, B J (1973) Resocializing the stroke patient . . . through a stroke club, Nursing Outlook, 21, Dec: 778-780

Ford, J (1971) Occupational therapy with stroke patients, Modern Geriatrics, 1: 414-422

Ordaei, D M and Walker, N S (1974) Group psychotherapy with stroke patients during the immediate recovery phase, American Journal of Orthopsychiatry, 44, April: 386-395

Oster, C and Kibat, W H (1975) Evaluation of a multidisciplinary care program in a day care centre, Journal of the American Geriatrics Society, 23, Feb: 63-69

Reed, D L (1970) Social disengagement in chronically ill patients, Nursing Research, 19: 109

Wasson, G F (1972) Volunteers assist stroke patients' recovery, Volunteer Leader, 13, June: 15-16

Whycherley, J (1974) Group therapy in the treatment of the hemiplegic patient, Nursing Mirror, 139 (6): 73-76

Sexuality

Berman, E and Lief, H I (1976) Sex and the ageing process, in W W Oakes (Editor) Sex and the Life Cycle, Grune & Stratton

Comfort, A (1974) Sexuality in old age, Journal of the American Geriatrics Society, 22, Oct: 440-442

Dean, S R (1974) Geriatric sexuality — normal, needed and neglected, Geriatrics, 29: 134-170

Friedman, J S (1978) Factors influencing sexual expression in the ageing process — a review of the literature, Journal of Psychiatric Nursing, 16, July: 34-47

Weinberg, J (1969) Sexual expression in later life, American Journal of Psychiatry, 126, Nov: 713-716

Woods Fugate, N (1975) Human Sexuality in Health and Illness, C V Mosby

Rehabilitation care

Ashley, P J (1970) Nursing aspects of rehabilitation, Nursing Times, 66 (35): 1102-1105

Brocklehurst, J C (1971) Guidelines for rehabilitating stroke patients — dysphagia and the nurse, Nursing Mirror, 133 (17): 17

Dolan, M B (1975) Re-thinking stroke — autumn months, autumn years, American

Journal of Nursing, 75, July: 1145-1147

Draper, J (1974) Long term care of the hemiplegic patient at home, Nursing Mirror, 139, Aug: 76-78

Elwood, E (1970) Nursing the patient with CVA, Nursing Clinics of North America, 5: 42

Fenwick, A M (1979) An interdisciplinary tool for assessing patients' readiness for discharge in the rehabilitation setting, Journal of Advanced Nursing, 4 (1): 9-23

Graham, L (1976) Stroke rehabilitation — a creative process, Canadian Nurse, 72, Feb: 22-28

Jay, P E (1980) Help Yourselves — A Handbook for Hemiplegics and Their Families, Butterworths

Kratz, C R (1975) Doctors, nurses and patients with stroke, Health, 12 (1), Spring: 16-18

Miller, C, Meier, R and Feldhausen, S (1974) Measurement of stroke care nursing proficiency, International Journal of Nursing Studies, 11: 211-222

Whitehouse, F A (1971) Stroke — the present challenge, Nursing Forum, 10 (1): 90-99

Williams, M E (1960) The patient profile, Nursing Research, 9 (3): 122-124

Wilkinson, M (1974) Treatment of hemiplegia in the acute stage, Nursing Mirror, 139 (6): 59-61

INDEX

LIPPINCOTT NURSING SERIES

The Lippincott Nursing Series is aimed specifically at meeting the needs of nurse education in the 1980s. New books, written by British nurses for British nurses, and adaptations of American texts reflect the ongoing changes in the profession of nursing. The Lippincott Nursing Series is essential reading for every nurse in training and practice.

Patient Related Multiple Choice Questions
Anne Betts, SRN, RNT, Senior Tutor; Cynthia Gilling, SRN, SCM, RNT, Assistant Director of Nurse Education; Marjorie Read, BA, SRN, RNT, DipN, Assistant Director of Nurse Education; Maureen Theobald, SRN, RCNT, RNT, DipEd. Senior Tutor, all at the Princess Alexandra School of Nursing, The London Hospital, London.

The Patient with a Respiratory Disorder
0 063182319   96 pp   paper   1982
The Patient with a Cardiovascular Disorder
0 06 318232 7   96 pp   paper   1982
The Patient with a Genitourinary Disorder
0 06 318253 X   96 pp   paper   August 1983

Handbook of Investigations
edited by Jennifer A Booth, SRN, SCM, RNT, DipEd, Senior Tutor (Postbasic Education), Macdonald Buchanan School of Nursing, The Middlesex Hospital, London
0 06318235 1   160 pp   paper   1982

The Lippincott Manual of Medical-Surgical Nursing
Lillian S Brunner, RN, MSN, ScD, FAAN, and Doris S Suddarth, RN, BSNE, MSN, Adapted for the UK

Volume 1: Total Patient Care; Rehabilitation Concepts; The Ageing Person; Care of the Surgical Patient; Emergency Nursing; Infectious Diseases; Care of the Patient with Cancer; Skin Disorders; Allergy Problems

0 06318207 6   418 pp   paper   December 1982

Volume 2: Conditions of the Cardiovascular System; Blood Disorders; Conditions of the Respiratory Tract; Disorders of the Digestive System; Metabolic and Endocrine Disorders

0 06 318208 4   512 pp   paper   December 1982

Volume 3: Conditions of the Nervous System; Ear Disorders; Eye Disorders; Musculoskeletal Conditions; Conditions of the Kidney, Urinary Tract and Reproductive System

0 06318209 2   418 pp   paper   December 1982

The Lippincott Manual of Paediatric Nursing
Lillian S Brunner, RN, MSN, ScD, FAAN, and Doris S Suddarth, RN, BSNE, MSN. Adapted for the UK by Barbara Weller, RSCN, SRN, RNT, Nursing Officer, DHSS; formerly Nurse Tutor, Hospital for Sick Children, Great Ormond Street and St Mary's Hospital, London

Physiology in Nursing
Marguerita Brunt, SRN, SCM, DipN, RCNT, RNT, Senior Tutor (Postbasic Education) Hammersmith Hospital, London
0 06 318227 0   196 pp   illus   1982

Geriatric Nursing
Charlotte Eliopoulos, RN, BS, MS
Adapted for the UK
0 06 318132 8   396 pp   paper   1980

SI Units for Nurses
John Glenn, formerly for Kesteven College, Grantham and David McCaugherty, SRN, RNT, School of Nursing, Princess Margaret Hospital, Swindon
School of Nursing, Princess Margaret Hospital, Swindon
0 06 318180 0   72 pp   paper   1981

Nursing the Patient in Pain
Margo McCaffery, RN, MS
Adapted for the UK by Beatrice Sofaer, BA, SRN, SCM, RCT, Nursing Research Unit, Department of Nursing Studies, University of Edinburgh
0 06 318239 4   448 pp   paper   April 1983

Nursing Care of the Hemiplegic Stroke Patient
Freda Myco, BA, SRN, BTS Cert, RNT, Lecturer, Department of Nursing
Studies, New University of Ulster, Northern Ireland
0 06 318248 3   224 pp   paper   May 1983

Communication for the Health Care Team
Voncile M Smith, PhD, and Thelma A Bass, MA
Adapted for the UK by Ann Faulkner, MA, DipEd, SRN, RCNT, Project
Director, Communication in Nurse Education (HEC Curriculum Develop-
ment Project), Department of Nursing, University of Manchester
0 06 318210 6   256 pp   paper   1982

Operating Theatre Nursing
Mary C Warren, SRN, RCNT, formerly Clinical Teacher, to the JBCNS
course in Operating Department Nursing, Charing Cross Hospital, London
0 06 318240 8   160 pp   paper   June 1983

Legal Problems in Nursing Practice
Ann Young, BA, SRN, RNT, Senior Tutor, Thomas Guy School of Nursing,
Guy's Hospital, London
0 06 318182 7   196 pp   paper   revised reprint April 1983